"We know the facts about thromboembolism. I think this is pretty uncontested. We know the facts about development of high blood pressure... We know the fact that certain patients get depressed on the pill. These are the facts we are all privy to."
- Alan Guttmacher, M.D.

"Birth control pills are dangerous and the public has not been given all the facts about them."
- Edmond Kassouf, M.D.

"I think they are to breast cancer what fertilizer is to the wheat crop."
- Roy Hertz, M.D.

"I believe that many of the women using the pill would switch to alternative methods if they knew the extent of the already-documented body pollution the pill is causing."
- Barbara Seaman

"It's staggering that for a drug that is being used by 80% of women, there is so little information about the long-term safety. That's really incredible."
- Ernst Rietzschel, M.D.

Only Dr. Rietzchel's quote is recent. The others came from leading researchers fifty years ago. Why is it that five decades later we still know so little about birth control safety?

Part One of this book explores the history, economics, and politics that gave us birth control before it was proven safe, and exposes the powerful forces working to keep us in the dark.

Part Two examines the myriad risks of hormonal birth control. From breast cancer and blood clots to depression and debilitating autoimmune disease, the health of millions of women has been sacrificed to chronic and deadly diseases **In the Name of The Pill**.

In the Name of
The Pill

Mike Gaskins

Copyright © 2019 Mike Gaskins

All rights reserved. No portion of this book may be reproduced or stored in a retrieval system by any means – electronic, mechanical, scanning, or other – except for brief quotations in critical reviews, articles, or related writings with proper citation, without the prior written permission of the publisher.

In the Name of The Pill/Mike Gaskins

Cover design by Leigh Finney, BirdhouseCreative.net

Paperback ISBN: 978-1-7337935-0-6

eBook ISBN: 978-1-7337935-1-3

*To my wife, Liz -
Without her support and encouragement, I never would have made it past this page.*

And to my daughters, Zoë and Gigi – Their energy and zest for life remind me every day why this fight is so important.

A Note on Structure

You may have picked up this book because you are interested in a specific health condition. For example, let's say you suffer from lupus. You've been curious about whether The Pill may have caused or contributed to your disease. Consequently, you may want to go directly to the chapter on lupus.

In an attempt to make pertinent information as accessible as possible, this book includes several chapters offering in-depth looks at individual diseases and how they have been linked to hormonal contraceptives. You will find those in Part Two. However, if that's where you choose to begin, you will probably find yourself with a lot of new questions. Most people do. Questions like:

"Why would my doctor give it to me if it wasn't safe?"

"How can experts say the benefits outweigh the risks?"

"Birth control has been on the market for decades. Why wouldn't they have taken it off the shelves if it's so dangerous?"

For the answers to those questions, you will want to start back from the beginning. The first part of the book focuses on the dynamics that originally brought The Pill to market and examines how those same forces actively protect its place in our current culture.

While my primary concern centers on the medical ramifications of hormonal birth control, no discussion on the topic would be complete without forays into the history, economics, and politics that gave us The Pill.

Of particular interest to the discussion is one unique moment in history - the Nelson Pill Hearings. These hearings, held in 1970 and chaired by Wisconsin Senator Gaylord Nelson, pulled back the curtains to reveal the powerful forces behind the legalization and promotion of birth control pills. The passing decades have not diminished the importance of the disturbing facts exposed in this little-known historical snapshot. The fact that these important hearings have largely been forgotten is a testament to the pharmaceutical industry's continuing influence and their efforts to control the message.

While this book is intended to encourage you to think critically about the medical advice you receive, it isn't meant to replace medical treatment or advice from a trained professional. If you think you need treatment or have symptoms related to any of the ailments discussed in this book, please schedule an appointment with the appropriate health care professional near you.

Part I – The Cause

1. A Responsibility to Tell	2
2. What They Knew	9
3. The Tide Begins to Turn	18
4. The Seminal Events	25
5. The Hearings Begin	32
6. Unsafe at Any Dose	42
7. A Greater Social Concern	55
8. The Dose Makes the Poison	75
9. The Green Plasma Mystery	80

Part II – The Effect

10. Migraines	94
11. More Deadly Blood Clots	100
12. Diabetes & Matters of the Heart	108
13. Birth Control & Breast Cancer	116
14. Permanent Sterilization	125
15. Depression and Mood Disorders	130
16. An Introduction to Autoimmune Disease	140
17. Systemic Lupus Erythematosus	146
18. Multiple Sclerosis	155
19. Crohn's Disease	159
20. Hair Was a Musical - Hair Loss Is a Drama	169
21. Thyroid, Liver, and Gallbladder	175
22. Something in the Water	184
23. How Do We Fix This Problem?	192

PART I
The Cause

In the Name of The Pill

CHAPTER 1

A Responsibility to Tell

Despite the overwhelming number of drugs on the market, there's only one pill known as *The* Pill.

The fanfare surrounding its introduction was grand. The country was in the midst of a cultural revolution that was changing the look and feel of everything.

For the first time, large groups of young people were protesting America's involvement in a foreign war. Flower children were calling for peace and love.

There was a move to replace natural products with what was being marketed as new and improved synthetic versions. Hardwood floors were covered up with bright laminated patterns and shag carpet. The breakfast table featured Tang instead of orange juice, and margarine instead of butter – so good it fooled Mother Nature.

And, a little miracle pill gave women hope that controlling their natural fertility could finally help level the playing field with men.

The Pill quickly moved from counter-cultural to mainstream, and today, it transcends fertility control, having grown into an iconic symbol of women's rights. It's difficult to have a conversation about The Pill without acknowledging its political significance.

Unfortunately, the political debate surrounding The Pill may be distracting us from the central issue of whether it's even safe for women to take.

Being Transparent

At the risk of being counter-cultural myself, I'd like to start off by being completely transparent. I'm a bald, middle-aged, Catholic man from Texas, who never quite outgrew being the class clown, and I'm passionate about The Pill.

You may be thinking, "Why is all that important?" And, honestly, I hope you are, because there are some people who think that at least three of those labels should disqualify me from having an opinion on The Pill (Four, if you count Texas against me). But, my passion for this subject is not driven by a moral or political agenda. I have no deep-seated desire to tell women what they should or shouldn't do. In fact, I have only one agenda – to expose the very real dangers of The Pill.

I feel it is important to tell you who I am up front because we live in a culture of extremes. We've lost the art of moderation. It seems we are all either Conservative or Liberal; Pro or Anti; Us or Them... Defined by extremes, there is no middle ground. Regardless of which side we're on, when someone offers a different perspective, we assume they are 'one of them.'

I never dreamed I would be a women's health advocate, but there's no denying that's what I've become.

My Distaste for The Pill

My distaste for The Pill predates any religion or spirituality in my life. For that matter, it also predates being bald, middle-aged, and Texan.

My wife and I were young and deeply in love. Somehow, that fact came up in a discussion with her doctor. She had gone in for something unrelated but came out with The Pill. That was fine with us. We hated condoms, and this sounded like the perfect solution. Since it had been on the market for decades, my wife never thought to question its safety.

One morning a few months in, I happened to be there as she opened a new package and the little patient-information booklet fell to the floor. Curiously, I picked it up and unfolded it. It felt like a hundred folds. Eventually, I got it open and began reading. I was horrified. "Honey, did the doctor mention any of these side effects to you?"

"What side effects?"

We sifted through the complicated text and discussed some of the warnings -- breast and cervical cancer, strokes, and heart disease. They were especially disconcerting given her family history. She asked whether the doctor would have given it to her if he thought it was dangerous.

Ultimately, it was a long, thoughtful conversation that ended with me saying, "I can't tell you what to do, but for me, if taking this pill means I get to spend even one less day with you at the end of our lives, it's not worth it."

It surprised me how much relief that statement brought her. She told me that the pills had been making her feel crazy and she immediately decided to stop taking them. Beyond my wife, my attitude about The Pill was indifferent. I never thought to ask my sisters if they had read the pamphlet or if their doctors had warned them. It didn't seem like my place.

Was it my place? Am I even allowed to talk about that with women beyond my wife? Where do my rights and responsibilities end?

Years passed. Then, a series of events brought me in contact with information that left me a little smarter than the average bear... at least where The Pill is concerned. That's when it occurred to me how few women were being given a fair chance to make a truly informed decision.

When you're privy to information that you *know* most women haven't been told about The Pill, does your responsibility change? I think it does. I have friends and relatives who suffered consequences because I didn't discuss The Pill with them sooner. I believe anyone who learns the truth about The Pill should act on the urge to share the information – to drown out the silence of doctors.

First Clue

As a writer and media producer, it was work that first inspired my Pill quest. Writing requires a natural curiosity. Whether I'm developing a video project or

A Responsibility to Tell

creating a marketing piece for a corporate client, I'm always looking for an interesting story.

A medical project in early 2015 brought me in contact with one of the world's leading authorities on autoimmune disease. I sat in on a meeting as this revered doctor spoke to a group of young specialists about the basics of the disease.

He told the group that they had known from the beginning that estrogen plays a crucial role in autoimmunity because nearly 80 percent of diagnoses are women and we know the role estrogen plays in a woman's immune system. He explained how estrogenic chemicals get into our system and mimic natural estrogens. They are known as endocrine disruptors.

My 'interesting story' radar went off even though it had nothing to do with the project at hand. I pulled out my phone. A quick Google search revealed that the incidence of many autoimmune diseases began climbing rapidly in the early 1970s.

I benefitted from limited knowledge. All I knew of the disease was a timeframe and what triggered it — chemicals mimicking natural estrogen. The only example I could think of was birth control pills. Based on what the good doctor had said, I assumed the connection must be well known in the medical community. I struck up a conversation with him after the meeting and asked exactly what role The Pill played in all of this. He replied, "None at all."

I was dumbfounded. "That seems impossible." I wasn't doubting him. In fact, I completely believed him regardless of how impossible it seemed. After all, he was the world-renowned authority.

He doubled down, "There hasn't been any evidence linking The Pill to autoimmunity."

The conversation continued for a while but didn't advance. It concluded with him saying, "Certainly, there are more questions than answers. And more research needs to be done."

I walked away feeling confused – as if the gentle old man had waved his hand and said, "These aren't the disruptors you're looking for."

That Nagging Feeling

I was still thinking about the encounter when I got back to my hotel room that evening. I pulled out my laptop and began my search with the first autoimmune disease that popped into my mind, "lupus + oral contraceptives." Among the top results was an article about a new study that found women who take The Pill are 50 percent more likely to develop lupus than nonusers.

I was thinking the famous doctor must be unaware of this new study. Then, halfway through the article, they had a quote from him. In black-and-white, the world-renowned authority I had just spoken with was telling women they shouldn't stop taking The Pill because of this study and that they needed to weigh the benefits against a 'very small increased risk of developing lupus.'

Had he lied to me? At best, he had undoubtedly played loose with the facts. Maybe he just thought it would be too deep for a simpleton like me and it was easier to say that no connection existed.

During the next few weeks, I continued my search and found numerous studies over several decades that linked The Pill to many autoimmune diseases. With each study, a pattern emerged. It seemed there was always a leading authority who was eager to say the benefits still outweighed the risks.

Questions About The Pill

Those initial searches left me with two burning questions that continue driving me to dig deeper for the truth:

1) Are doctors being forthright with women about birth control so that they can make truly informed decisions?
2) Why is the medical community always eager to downplay studies that find risks associated with hormonal contraceptives?

Though they aren't mutually exclusive, the two questions reflect the natural duality of The Pill. The first question deals primarily with the medical phenomenon of The Pill, while the second deals more with the social implications.

The answers to these questions can only begin to be understood by exploring the unique intersection of social, medical, and political forces that gave us this 'magic pill.'

CHAPTER 2

What They Knew

"What did they know, and when did they know it?"

From the time Howard Baker first uttered this infamous question of President Nixon during the Watergate scandal, it was destined to become a cliché that would underscore every future political scandal. Cliché or not, it is a valid question when it comes to the dangers of birth control. As we will see, there were *JAMA* warnings about synthetic estrogens dating back as far as 1940. We have to wonder what the leaders of both political parties knew and when they knew it. The unfortunate answer is they knew a lot, and even if they weren't familiar with the *JAMA* warnings, they certainly knew about the dangers in great detail by the time the Nelson Pill Hearings concluded in 1970.

Opening a Can of Worms

January 14, 1970 was a typically cold winter morning in Washington D.C. As Senator Gaylord Nelson and his top staffer, Ben Gordon, walked to Capitol Hill, they were confronted by protestors. Groups of women walked alongside them yelling their disapproval. Their breath rose visibly through the air, creating the impression they were literally venting steam.

It was the age of Peace, Love, and Happiness but these women were protesting something much more important than the frivolity of the sexual revolution. They saw The Pill as a tool that would allow them to control their fertility - it enabled them to plan their families around their careers. Skeptical of the male-dominated Senate, they saw this attack on The Pill as a power grab — an attempt to remove their chance for equality.

The hearings were controversial before they had even begun.

I was fortunate enough to have the chance to become friends with Ben Gordon later in his life, after being introduced to him by Morton Mintz (more on both of these gentlemen in coming pages). In a recent conversation, Mr. Gordon recalled that most of the early protesters were upset because they felt that the senators might have a hidden agenda for going after birth control. However, as the hearings progressed and leading physicians shared their concerns about The Pill's safety, the outcry from protestors shifted. They began to question why they were being used as guinea pigs by the drug companies.

Today, decades later, the hearings have largely been forgotten. But, because so many women continue to be affected by this potent medication, the information revealed in the hearings is more relevant than ever. It may provide the only snapshot in history, where the inner workings of the pharmaceutical industry were so clearly revealed. Testimony linked The Pill to everything from cancer, heart disease, and strokes, to lupus, depression, and diabetes - facts that had previously been (and continue to be) obfuscated by Big Pharma. Beyond side effects and complications, the hearings exposed an astounding and far-reaching abuse of power. The industry commonly flexed its muscles to manipulate the FDA, influence research, and intimidate the media, and there is no reason to believe things have changed in today's world.

Like any pivotal moment in history, there is a vibrant backstory.

Borne of Rage

Young Margaret Sanger was nineteen years old when her mother died of tuberculosis. She blamed her mother's early demise on having birthed eleven children and miscarried seven others. She channeled the rage from her mother's death toward a new inspiration - a vision to develop a 'magic pill' that would prevent unwanted pregnancies.

After decades of frustrating fights over fertility laws and ineffective contraceptives, her passion was refueled by a growing focus on overpopulation and population control. In 1951, she met Dr. Gregory Pincus, a man she believed could bring her dream to reality. Collectively, they ignored the many warnings about the dangers of synthetic estrogens. Their collaboration soon showed enough promise to garner support from the biggest names in corporate America, including the Rockefellers, the Ford Foundation, and Shell Oil – all names that were already active in the fight for population control.

Eager to advance their agenda, Katharine McCormick, heiress to the International Harvester fortune, lamented in a letter to Margaret Sanger, "[We need] a cage of ovulating females to experiment with."

They found their 'cage' in the slums of Puerto Rico.

Puerto Rico Trials

Backed by the deepest pockets in the United States, a group of doctors brought their 'magic pill' to Puerto Rico in 1956, promising women it 'would keep them from having children they couldn't support.' However, the women weren't informed that they were actually participating in a trial for a powerful and under-researched drug. Nor were they warned of potential side effects.

The entire trial was riddled with dubious and deceitful practices, which still hang like a dark cloud over the island. Ray Quintanilla, a journalist for The Orlando Sentinel, visited Puerto Rico in 2004, fifty years after the trials began. He discovered that time had yet to heal the wounds. Bitter feelings still simmered about the secrecy and experimental nature of those events. He spoke with tearful women who participated in the trial, and still questioned why they were not allowed to make decisions for themselves. They told him the story of how these doctors from the US showed up in white lab coats to deliver their babies but were soon recruiting them to try The Pill.

The bitter feelings aren't just about having placed their trust in deceptive doctors. On a deeper level, the villagers realize they were unwitting guinea pigs used to test a potent and dangerous drug. In fact, five seemingly healthy participants died during the trial. They were buried without an autopsy, and their deaths were never attributed to the medication.

It's interesting to note, when 'credible' sources write about the Puerto Rico pill trials today, they typically cite that either two or three women died in the trials (if they mention the deaths at all). However, at the Nelson Pill Hearings, the undisputed number of deaths was five. It's as if the facts of the narrative have been rewritten over time.

A Troubled FDA

Thanks to impeccable timing The Pill met virtually no resistance on its path to FDA approval as a contraceptive. The sexual revolution had just crossed paths with fears of a looming population explosion. People everywhere were excited about the promises of a pill that could control the number of births. Consequently, the focus was on The Pill's efficacy rather than its safety.

The Food and Drug Administration of the late 1950s and early 1960s bore little resemblance to the FDA we know today. In those days, the agency lacked the power to hold drug manufacturers accountable. Federal investigators relied heavily on the evidence presented to them by industry researchers.

Dr. Pincus' group presented selective results from their Puerto Rico trial to the FDA just as the William S. Merrell drug company petitioned the agency to approve another drug as a treatment for morning sickness during pregnancy. Though Thalidomide would never be approved, it forever changed the FDA and this country's drug approval process.

Enovid, the first formulation of birth control pill, was quickly approved for contraceptive use mere months before the Thalidomide scandal exploded. Thalidomide was already being used throughout Europe, and the Merrell company distributed samples across the United States while they awaited approval. Fortunately, a brave young Pharmacology Ph.D. who had only been with the FDA for a month was assigned to review the application. Dr. Frances O. Kelsey found it unsettling that there was a lack of evidence surrounding the drug's safety in humans. She was also disturbed by the behavior of the petitioning company, saying that she felt they were never frank with her throughout the process.

Dr. Kelsey stood by her convictions despite the drug company's attempts to strong-arm her. By early 1962, it became widely known that the drug was causing atrocious birth defects throughout Europe. The United States had been spared the devastating consequences of Thalidomide, and Dr. Kelsey was lauded as a national hero -- thanks in large part to the reporting of Morton Mintz in the Washington Post.

He broke the story in the Sunday paper, July 15, 1962:

"This is the story of how the skepticism and stubbornness of a Government physician prevented what could have been an appalling American tragedy, the birth of hundreds or indeed thousands of armless and legless children.

"The story of Dr. Frances Oldham Kelsey, a Food and Drug Administration medical officer, is not one of inspired prophecies nor of dramatic research breakthroughs.

"She saw her duty in sternly simple terms, and she carried it out, living the while with insinuations that she was a bureaucratic nitpicker, unreasonable – even, she said, stupid...

"What she did was refuse to be hurried into approving an application for marketing a new drug."

After refusing to be bullied into approving the dangerous drug, Dr. Kelsey received the President's Award for Distinguished Federal Civilian Service from John F. Kennedy, and her tenacious stand started a domino effect that led to monumental changes at the FDA.

Uncovering the Ineptitude

Questions and concerns about the FDA and drug regulation had already been moving into the forefront of public awareness, but the Thalidomide scandal brought them to a head. Congress reacted by passing the Kefauver-Harris Drug Amendments, which gave the FDA more control over the approval process and required the drug companies to report adverse reactions. Though too late for the women who suffered through the Puerto Rico experiment, the new legislation required companies to inform patients they were participating in a trial and obtain their consent before proceeding.

Senator Hubert Humphrey, who was a pharmacist before becoming a politician, turned up the heat even more by launching a subcommittee to investigate ineptitude at the FDA. This investigation revealed that Enovid had been approved based on only 132 women taking The Pill for 12 consecutive months! Writing for the Columbia Journalism Review this time, Morton Mintz was again on the story. Noting that some women may take this powerful drug for 30 years, he was appalled by the small sample size and duration of the trial. He concluded:

> "As a basis for presuming safety in long-term use by, ultimately millions of women, this was a scientific scandal... For one thing, 132 is a smaller number of women than, this year alone, will die from clotting induced by The Pill."

Timing Is Everything

Studying the early timeline of The Pill is like watching an action movie filled with near misses. So many times the dangers of The Pill could have and should have been caught, but then, at just the right moment, forces would align to buoy its progress. In some cases, these forces were engineered. Others could be attributed to good timing. Yet in many cases, it's difficult to discern what was manipulation and what was chance.

The FDA approved The Pill based on insufficient data just months before the Thalidomide scandal changed everything. Then, an investigative Congressional Subcommittee discovered that the trial upon which the approval had been based involved an indefensibly small sample size. Their findings hit the headlines as 'a scientific scandal.' The Pill's safety concerns began to loom larger in the public consciousness.

This was the cliffhanger moment. It looked like The Pill was in trouble. However, just when it seemed the magic pill was backed into an impossible corner, Lyndon

B. Johnson chose Sen. Humphrey to be his Vice Presidential running mate in the 1964 election. Quietly, the special subcommittee headed by Sen. Humphrey was aborted, and the headlines it generated would be forgotten soon enough.

One can't help but wonder how different things would have been if Dr. Pincus' team had submitted their findings just a few months later - after the Thalidomide scandal. In a 1967 appearance on Face the Nation, the new FDA Commissioner, James Goddard M.D., suggested the fate of The Pill could have been very different. Once again, it was Morton Mintz digging for answers.

As a frequent guest journalist on the program, Mr. Mintz developed a reputation for his hard-hitting questions. He raised the issue of the small trial size and duration (132 women for 12 months) and asked Commissioner Goddard if he believed this was adequate scientific foundation to approve The Pill. Goddard said that he had been under the impression that large-scale studies had preceded the approval process. Here's how Mr. Mintz recalls what happened next, "Then a huge TV audience across America heard him say: 'Whether today, if the same problem came up de novo, I would make the same judgment that was made then, I can't say.'"

In the end, Margaret Sanger finally got her magic pill. However, the problem with magic is that it is based on illusion, and the truth is often obscured.

CHAPTER 3

The Tide Begins to Turn

The Pill was entangled in a web of uncertainty within its first decade on the market and clotting issues were the biggest concern. Doctors throughout the nation were reporting cases of young women suffering and sometimes dying from strokes and emboli. Despite mounting evidence, the drug manufacturers refused to take responsibility for the grave complications. Rather, they employed a public relations strategy to cast doubt on the findings. Ironically, they claimed the sample size was too small to draw any conclusions and that more research needed to be done.

The resulting hesitation to discuss The Pill's drawbacks frustrated leading physicians who felt they were just beginning to uncover the dangers. Dr. David Clark, a world-renowned neurologist, lamented that it was as if The Pill had been granted a sort of "diplomatic immunity."

The British Invade

Concerns about The Pill's safety continued to surface, but drug makers managed to contain the damage until April 1968. That's when the British Medical Journal released the results of the Inman-Vessey mortality study, a retrospective study that demonstrated a 7.5-fold increased risk of death from stroke in young women taking The Pill.

The study was sufficiently large, scientifically sound, replicable, and the news was devastating. The dangers of hormonal birth control could no longer be ignored. Of course, many of the doctors who had been defending The Pill all along continued to support it, downplaying the risks. Some doctors had achieved a level of fame defending The Pill. These same players hit the media circuit in an attempt to minimize the damage. But this time, things felt different. Previously, some might have wondered if these doctors were shills for the drug companies, but now there was little doubt.

One celebrity doctor, Dr. Louis Hellman was the Chairman of the FDA advisory board that was supposed to have investigated The Pill's safety. While on his media parade, he stopped by the Today Show to tell viewers that the risk was "very, very small," and reassured them that The Pill "has proved remarkably safe."

The Torchbearers

On a broader scale, the British study inspired a new breed of hero. The seeds of enlightenment began with three people. A doctor, a reporter, and a feminist commenced the arduous task of bringing to light the dangers of this medication. In 1969, each of them published books on the topic.

Harold Williams M.D.: The Doctor

Dr. Harold Williams was a physician and practicing attorney who felt it was time for someone from the medical community to speak up about the dangers of The Pill. Here's how he described the political climate in the liner notes of his book, *Pregnant or Dead*, "Much of the medical profession and the public have become polarized into pro-Pill and anti-Pill factions. Only the proponents have been well organized and well financed. So far, they have held the upper hand…"

Using available science and vital statistics, Dr. Williams demonstrated how mortality rates in young women had shifted in the few short years since birth control had been introduced. His 'conservative estimate' was that an additional 850 young women were dying in the U.S. from vascular disorders each year - and this was before The Pill had even reached critical mass.

You can sense the underlying anger as Dr. Williams describes the strategy used by the drug companies to deny the medication's link to serious clotting issues:

"So long as the data presented could be claimed as 'the best available' there was a ready-made defense for any hiatus in the data. As long as The Pill proponents expressed a desire for more complete data – all the while taking steps to thwart its compilation – they were safe…Then came the British. They reported preliminarily that a well-planned study was showing a distinctly higher incidence of thromboembolic disasters among Pill-takers... This required some new strategy. Now it became necessary to try to discredit the British work, and at the same time to continue stalling studies in the United States that might yield similar results."

Perhaps even more shocking were the results when Dr. Williams compiled statistics for another (less discussed) side effect. Recognizing that depression was one of the most common complaints, he reviewed suicide statistics from the most recent year (1967) and compared them with statistics from 1961 (representing the last year before birth control became commonplace). He found that the suicide rate among young women from the ages of 15 to 24 had nearly doubled.

These increases were dramatically higher than their male counterparts. By extension, Dr. Williams had shown that the collateral damage from birth control could be much broader than most skeptics first considered.

Morton Mintz: The Reporter

As the medical reporter for the *Washington Post*, Morton Mintz won many prestigious awards for his previously mentioned reports on birth defects caused by Thalidomide. In 1965, he turned his attention to The Pill. His dispassionate, 'Just the facts, ma'am' approach reflected a journalistic integrity not motivated by any political agenda.

The authenticity of Mr. Mintz's work resulted from a genuine desire to be able to say The Pill had been proven safe. In the introduction to his book, *The Pill: An Alarming Report*, Mr. Mintz explained that he and his wife were members of Planned Parenthood, and, "Nothing could have pleased me more than to have found that The Pill was free of hazards. However, the answers made it overwhelmingly clear that safety had not been established."

When I contacted Mr. Mintz while researching this book, he began the conversation with a caveat: "I'm 93 and have forgotten mountains of stuff."

However, the mountains of stuff he remembered were fascinating. He said that, as a reporter, he had no opinion of whether The Pill was safe or unsafe. "What concerned me was the stunning inadequacy of the evidence of safety that the FDA had in hand when it approved The Pill."

I asked him about his exchange with FDA Commissioner Robert Goddard on *Face the Nation* when the commissioner admitted that the evidence had been insufficient. This was a stunning admission that Mr. Mintz recalled fondly, "I was invited on such shows to challenge the likes of the Commissioner of the FDA and the chairman of Philip Morris with, I egotistically thought, wonderful results."

Mr. Mintz was the only major press member to stay on the story once the headlines began to fade. He continued to report on The Pill until 1977 when his bosses abruptly moved him back to covering the Supreme Court. He later learned from a friend at the *New York Times* that he had been reassigned because a well-connected woman at the *Washington Post* had gone to the editor, Ben Bradlee, and said she was "sick and tired" of Mort's stories on The Pill because "...she and her friends used it and knew it was safe." Her anecdotal 'proof' was apparently enough to have the final committed journalist taken off the beat.

Barbara Seaman: The Feminist

Barbara Seaman's passionate investigation of synthetic estrogens began as a young woman after her Aunt Sally died of uterine cancer at the age of 49, presumably from taking Premarin, a first generation synthetic hormone replacement therapy derived from horse urine.

After her death, the doctor warned the women in the family that they should never take such drugs. However, when the lure of birth control pills came along, the young Ms. Seaman didn't immediately make the connection. She was a young, driven, politically active member of the women's equality movement and a perfect candidate for The Pill. Without so much as a second thought, she began to take birth control. Like many women, it took a while for Ms. Seaman to connect her unpleasant side effects to The Pill. She had started losing hair - so much so that she grew concerned that she might be going bald in her twenties. She visited many doctors about the dramatic hair loss, and none of them considered birth control a potential culprit. Eventually, it was Ms. Seaman who pieced together the timing of her problems and attributed them to The Pill.

That experience lent credence to the earlier warning from her aunt's doctor. Together, these events inspired her to build a career fighting synthetic hormones and the "Don't worry your pretty little head" mentality that she had witnessed in the medical industry. She continued the mission until her death in 2008. Along the way, she learned that many prominent physicians shared her concerns about The Pill.

Her first book, *The Doctors' Case Against The Pill*, combined scientific research with personal stories from the perspective of doctors and women who had encountered problems with The Pill.

A Collective Rumble

Collectively, these three books sparked a national conversation. Women began to question The Pill's safety and were no longer taking prescriptions on blind faith. For the first time, there seemed to be a formidable pushback against the pharmaceutical marketing machine.

CHAPTER 4

The Seminal Events

It was a rather unceremonious beginning to what would become the longest running Congressional hearings in our nation's history. On a mid-May morning in 1967, members of the Select Committee on Small Business gathered in room 318 of the Old Senate Office Building. The title of the hearings was intentionally broad, *Competitive Problems in the Drug Industry*. The chairman of the committee, Senator Gaylord Nelson intended the hearings to be a thorough investigation of the drug companies and their business practices.

Thorough they were. It would take just over a decade before the gavel came down on the final session of the hearings, eclipsing The Truman Hearings by a full three years. The Truman Hearings ran from 1941-1948 and investigated the role of private business in World War II, working to protect the defense department from war profiteering. Truman's hearings are often mistakenly cited as the longest running hearings in Congressional history. However, the war and its hearings were finite, while the ambitious drug hearings seemed to have endless source material. These hearings examined a vast range of issues in the drug industry (most of which are ripe to be revisited today), including questionable pricing practices, deceptive advertising, safety and efficacy of over-the-counter products, generics versus name brands, rebranding and marketing of products proven unsafe... Ultimately, the hearings would fill thirty-three volumes in the Congressional Library.

As they progressed, the hearings garnered their share of attention in the press. Occasionally, they would lead off the evening news or appear above the fold in the *Washington Post* and *New York Times*, but nothing in the hearings compared to the firestorm that hit in early 1970 when the committee turned its attention to birth control. This relatively small sample of the overall hearings took on a life of its own, and would forever be known as the Nelson Pill Hearings.

A Letter to the Senator

In her book, Barbara Seaman intertwined compelling science on the dangers of The Pill with emotional anecdotal stories from some of the women subjected to the consequences. She expected their stories to spark a national outrage, but the book hadn't received as much attention as she had hoped.

Aware of the drug industry hearings that were taking place on Capitol Hill, Ms. Seaman saw the symbiotic possibilities and penned a six-page letter to Sen. Nelson outlining some of her gravest concerns. Here are some key excerpts from that letter:

"Never before in history have so many millions of people taken such a powerful and unnecessary drug."

"You cannot long knock any natural system out of balance without doing some harm - whether it shows up immediately or years later. Furthermore, many of these pill-caused metabolic disturbances are progressive. The longer a woman stays on the pill, the more her laboratory tests are altered."

"I believe that many of the women using the pill would switch to alternative methods if they knew the extent of the already-documented body pollution the pill is causing."

"Why has the suggestive evidence about the two most frightening possibilities – cancer and genetic damage, been generally withheld from the public, including physicians?"

She bolstered her argument with quotes from revered physicians like Dr. Harry Rudel, one of the developers of The Pill, who admitted: "The pill is something we entered into with the best of faith, something we truly believed affected only ovulation and fertility. It was a relatively small dose of a drug, and it appeared that it was not affecting anything except fertility. Then as we began to look, we began to see that we are influencing many systems in the body."

A quote she included from Dr. Philip Corfman of the National Institutes of Health may have been the most damning. He said, "There is no organ or system of the body which, upon examination, has not been found to be affected by the pill."

Now That I Have Your Attention

Ms. Seaman had more in common with the senator than she imagined. They both believed they had uncovered some seriously unscrupulous problems with the pharmaceutical industry, and that these critical discoveries had gone largely unnoticed by the public. It is always difficult to gauge when the media is driving public attention versus when public interest begins to drive media coverage, but Sen. Nelson knew he needed a hot-button topic if his hearings were going to generate appropriate publicity.

Ms. Seaman's letter hit its mark. Sen. Nelson passed it along to his lead staffer, Ben Gordon and asked him to look into making it part of their hearings. Mr. Gordon had spent ten years on Capitol Hill prior to working with Sen. Nelson, and the senator trusted him implicitly.

Most congressional hearings throughout history have been staffed by a team that coordinates and manages the hearings, but Mr. Gordon was a one-man band. He assembled the roster of experts to testify at the hearings, wrote the opening statements, and did all of the extensive legwork behind the scenes. Throughout the proceedings, he sat at the table next to Chairman Nelson and frequently chimed in with questions and comments. Consequently, it may have been just as important that the letter resonated with Mr. Gordon as it had with the senator – and it did. Mr. Gordon eagerly set up a meeting with Ms. Seaman.

With Sen. Nelson passing away in 2005, Mr. Gordon is one of the few living people who can give a first-person account of the inner workings of the hearings. When I started speaking with the reporter, Morton Mintz, about my research on The Pill, he said, "You know who you should talk to - Ben Gordon. He's 102-years-old but still sharp as a tack."

If anything, Mr. Mintz may have underestimated how sharp Mr. Gordon was! I was amazed by the lucid memories he was able to share with me. At one point, he stopped to say, "The drug companies are a bunch of bastards, and you can quote me on that... Not really, but they *are* a bunch of bastards." Figuring he had nothing to lose, he later gave me permission to quote him (lest you think I dishonored the request of a 102-year-old man).

He told me about his first meeting with Ms. Seaman and how he initially thought he would call her to testify. However, upon reading the research in her book, he decided it would be better to go with the doctors whose studies she cited. He said he has always had a policy to avoid indirect testimony because it is too easily picked apart. He added that, as he spoke with these respected physicians, he was surprised to learn that many doctors felt as if The Pill was being forced upon them by the drug industry.

The Iceberg Beneath

Before the hearings, if a woman heard about complications related to The Pill, it was likely to be about either breast cancer or thrombosis. Shockwaves rippled across the country as the hearings revealed the iceberg that lurked beneath the surface. Suddenly, women were hearing world-renowned physicians talk about complications that seemed impossibly diverse – lupus, diabetes, suicide, strokes, libido, hair loss, arthritis, migraines, sterility, as well as negative impacts on metabolism, weight, skin, and vision.

Even a cursory review of the hearings decades later shows the wisdom of Mr. Gordon's decision to go with direct testimony from the doctors who had conducted the studies. Senator Bob Dole from Kansas was particularly nasty to any doctor who suggested The Pill had safety issues. According to Mr. Gordon, "Dole was on our committee, and when he came, there was no question he was representing the industry." And the transcripts suggest Sen. Dole had little interest in hiding his bias.

As proud as he is of the hearings, Mr. Gordon admits he is surprised that no other politician has 'taken up the torch.' Unfortunately, news reporters have dropped the ball as well. When I asked Mr. Mintz whether he thought today's journalists shared his sense of duty to protect citizens, he replied, "Have you ever seen an editorial condemning corporate misconduct other than financial shenanigans? I can't recall any."

It would be natural at this point to think, "It's been 50 years! Surely, today's version of The Pill has been proven safe."

That's a reasonable assumption. However, it's dead wrong. The maker of today's most popular birth control brands, Yaz and Yasmin, paid out $2.04 billion to settle over 10,000 blood-clot lawsuits as of January 2016, and the number of injuries, deaths, and lawsuits continues to rise.

The truth behind Dr. Corfman's statement remains, "There is no organ or system of the body which, upon examination, has not been found to be affected by the pill."

Yet, our politicians and journalists are no longer interested in the conversation. The modern debate about birth control availability and its place in health care overshadow the larger and more fundamental issue of whether it is even safe.

It seems as though we have forgotten that these are in fact powerful medications - synthetic chemicals with serious side effects. It is these side effects that bridge the past and the present. In page after dusty page of the decades-old hearings, there is an alarming amount of prophetic testimony. Many of the 'rare' complications doctors were attributing to The Pill at the hearings are manifested in large numbers today.

Prophets are typically considered heretical by their contemporaries but are revered by future generations once the truth of their prophecies is revealed. Up until now, the prophets from these hearings have been silenced and buried by the efforts of the pharmaceutical industry's massive public relations machine.

Millions of women, young and old, still suffer the consequences of this suppressed information. It's time to reconsider these hearings in light of their relevance to the plight of women today – women whose complications range from depression to chronic disease and even death.

CHAPTER 5

The Hearings Begin

It didn't take long for the hearings to captivate the nation. Women watched in horror, shocked to hear researchers discuss the many potential dangers of birth control. They heard leading authorities admit that no one really knew the ramifications, but that it could take decades to see the full impact. Women across the country began to panic. Doctors' offices were inundated with phone calls from women demanding answers.

Pill proponents grew indignant, including Sen. Dole, who claimed, "There must be certain advantages to the pill other than avoiding pregnancy. I think we probably have terrified a number of women around the country... I would guess they may be taking two pills now – first a tranquilizer and then the regular pill – because of our erudite investigation."

Sen. Nelson calmly retorted that if the women had been told about the dangers of The Pill *before* being prescribed, then they wouldn't be alarmed hearing about them now.

Indeed, millions of women suddenly found themselves feeling betrayed by the medical establishment. Their dismay paved the way for new alliances in the burgeoning women's health movement.

Much like Barbara Seaman, whose book ultimately inspired the hearings, Alice Wolfson experienced dramatic hair loss when she began taking The Pill. Both women were assured by multiple doctors that birth control wasn't causing their hair loss, and each came to the conclusion, on her own, that indeed it was. The nonchalant attitude of their doctors inspired them to push back against a system that didn't seem to care.

At the hearings, Alice Wolfson became a familiar face. In fact, she became *the* original face of the women's health movement after she famously interrupted the hearings to question why 10 million women were being used as guinea pigs.

Ms. Seaman met with Ms. Wolfson after her outburst, and they became fast friends. Ms. Seaman later wrote about the hearings saying it brought the "uptown" and "downtown" feminists together on the issue of birth control safety. She and Ms. Wolfson would go on to found the National Women's Health Network. To this day, it is one of the nation's top women's health advocacy groups.

Doctors Not on Board

It also became apparent, for the first time in the public arena that not all doctors were on board with hormonal birth control. Some of them weren't comfortable with the idea of birth control in general and others weren't keen on prescribing a drug to 'treat' a normal process. As Dr. Herbert Ratner explained in his testimony, "This is the first time in medicine's history the drug industry has placed at our disposal a powerful, disease-producing chemical for use in the healthy rather than the sick."

As proof, he referred to two reports, which revealed that twenty to fifty percent of women on The Pill reported complications. He warned there would be a sharp rise in 'physician-caused disease.' Doctor after doctor expressed similar concerns. Dr. John Laragh said, "Sometimes 8 or 10 years go by before a very serious side effect is appreciated... this is a mass population experiment in this sense." Dr. Philip Ball referred to it as 'internal pollution by chemicals.' Even Dr. Alan Guttmacher, the president of Planned Parenthood/World Population advised, "The physician should be made to understand and appreciate that unless he can see the patient who is on the pill at least every 6 months, he should not prescribe it for her."

Many doctors familiar with the research were beginning to see that drug makers had done everything they could to control the message reaching the medical industry at large. They had manipulated studies and reported selective findings. Generally, they had worked to obfuscate any and all bad news related to The Pill. That is precisely why the hearings were so shocking.

The hearings exposed their dubious practices, but it also provided a glimpse into how much broader the cover-up was. In his testimony, Dr. Edmond Kassouf outlined the pharmaceutical industry's many devious tactics to engineer a positive message about their miracle pill. One piece of evidence he pointed to was the *New York Times* negative review of Barbara Seaman's book, *The Doctors' Case Against The Pill*. The reviewer wrote, "One wonders why the drug companies have been so exercised by it. In a way, their attempts to warn book reviewers against it are more disturbing than the book itself."

Dr. Kassouf marveled, "[The reviewer] has performed a public service in exposing the drug companies' attempts [to bury the book]."

But, the drug companies' attempts didn't stop at squelching book reviews. In the 25th anniversary edition of her book, Ms. Seaman, who also wrote for *Ladies Home Journal*, *Good Housekeeping*, and *Bride's Magazine*, described how all of her regular outlets let her go. One of the editors admitted that an ad agency for one of the drug companies had approached them about a seven-and-a-half-million-dollar campaign for a new diaper-rash ointment, but expressed concern that Ms. Seaman was damaging sales for an important prescription drug from that same drug maker.

She was eventually picked up by the *New York Times* in 1975. As the successful author of two books, they offered her scale. Ms. Seaman questioned why she would be making half of what they were paying their food writer, adding, "her job is fun; mine would be hard." The editor replied, "Yes, but she would bring in ads, and you will lose them."

Decades have passed, but the tactics employed by the drug companies were so successful, it would be foolish to think this doesn't happen today – especially in light of the fact that their advertising budgets have broadened exponentially to include prescription medications.

Beyond the Medicine

After years of nothing but Pleasantville news about The Pill, the Nelson Pill Hearings must have felt like a horror movie marathon to medical professionals and their young patients taking birth control. Years of cover-up and 'whitewashing of evidence' gave way to a series of truthful revelations about the gigantic dangers attached to the harmless looking little pill.

One physician submitted a portion of a booklet produced by *Child and Family* magazine, entitled *The Medical Hazards of the Birth Control Pill*. The booklet contended that the drug makers acted less like an industry concerned about the public welfare, and more like big business concerned only with profits. The authors didn't mince words when they wrote:

> "Drug manufacturers began to manipulate professional opinion at an early date, stressing the wonders of The Pill and minimizing its dangers. In this they were aided by medical journalists, who for a long time – with a few exceptions – filed "gee-whiz" stories that tended to condition lay readers to a positive orientation toward oral contraceptives."

Testimony at the hearings inspired a completely different kind of "gee whiz" reaction. More like, "Gee whiz, could they have been any more devious?" This wasn't just a medical issue, and it wasn't just a women's issue; it was a major news story competing with the likes of the Vietnam War and desegregation in the south.

Viewers who previously hadn't given The Pill a second thought were suddenly confronted with very stark realities.

Perhaps just as disturbing as the warnings about side effects and complications were the experts who testified as proponents of The Pill. They all offered disclaimers or spoke in mitigating terms, as we saw with Dr. Guttmacher's warning that a patient should be seen every six months. Meanwhile, Dr. Mary Lane from the Margaret Sanger Research Bureau suggested the follow-up should actually be as short as every four months.

It also became evident in the hearings that these doctors never intended for The Pill to be used as anything more than a way to create space between children. Several doctors warned that The Pill should never be taken for longer than two years. The unknown dangers of extended use were just too unpredictable. In fact, Dr. Roy Hertz from the Population Council stated, "The application of these medications in their present state of knowledge constitutes a highly experimental undertaking. That the individual called upon to take these materials, particularly for a prolonged period of time, should be regarded as, in effect, a volunteer for an experimental undertaking. I think she should be so informed."

Everyone knew the patients *weren't* being informed, and, for many who testified, that was the issue. They saw the introduction of The Pill as a philosophical dilemma harkening back to Aristotle, who had warned that 'effective drugs given to the healthy are bound to lead to imbalance and disease.'

The First Signs of Trouble

Hormonal birth control is not natural. The estrogens in them are not natural. They are synthetic chemicals that mimic natural estrogen in order to trick the healthy body into thinking it is pregnant, thereby preventing actual pregnancy. This is as true today as it was in 1970 when Dr. Hugh Davis said this in his testimony that opened the hearings, "To think of them as natural is comforting but quite false."

Many doctors began sounding the alarms early. They witnessed 'imbalance and disease' caused by The Pill in the form of strokes among young women. As we've already seen, the industry denied there was any link until the British study forced them to change their tune. Most discussion of specific diseases will come in the second half of this book, but the subject of strokes provides an excellent opportunity to scrutinize how the industry molded the conversation from the beginning, and how the perspective has (or hasn't) evolved over time.

Testimony Without Equivocation

The science linking birth control pills to strokes hasn't changed. No one has seriously disputed the correlation since *The Lancet* first published Dr. Wynn's study in 1966.

Pay attention to this excerpt from Dr. Alan Guttmacher's testimony, keeping in mind he was the founding president of Planned Parenthood/World Population:

> "We know the facts about thromboembolism. I think this is pretty uncontested. We know the facts about

development of high blood pressure in a certain small proportion of patients. We know the fact that certain patients get depressed on the pill. These are the facts we are all privy to."

Earlier in the hearings, Dr. J. Edwin Wood explained the phenomenon of strokes appearing in healthy young women this way:

"One of the major contributing causes of thrombosis in veins appears to be that of reduced velocity of flow of blood in the veins or relative stagnation or stasis of flow in the veins...
"Studies of women taking oral contraceptive agents have led to the clear-cut finding of dilatation of the veins of the extremities – other veins as well perhaps but they have not been studied. These dilated veins carry the same amount of blood as before, but since they are wider in diameter the blood flows more slowly.
"The net effect of this series of events is a slowing of the blood flow during oral contraceptive therapy."

Clearly, the facts about hormonal contraceptives and strokes were well known in 1970, yet they somehow still escape the curriculum in today's medical schools.

Not-So-Wild Conspiracy Theory

Is it really possible that the drug industry actively worked for the past fifty years to keep the dangers of birth control out of the public consciousness? Even for those who might be inclined to skepticism, one major headline from late 2017 certainly made the idea seem plausible.

The Hearings Begin

A damning investigative report from Reuters revealed that Johnson and Johnson, a major birth control manufacturer, knew about safety issues with another of its iconic products, Johnson's Baby Powder, as far back as 1957. The talc used in their baby powder comes from underground mines, and very often, veins of asbestos run through those talc deposits. Asbestos is a dangerous carcinogen, and for some people, even relatively low exposures can lead to mesothelioma or ovarian cancer.

As part of an ongoing lawsuit, J&J was forced to turn over tomes of internal documents to plaintiff's attorneys who claimed the company knew about the presence of asbestos and its dangers, yet failed to protect their consumers. It's worth reviewing this tangent because many of the tactics revealed in the internal memos parallel tactics used by the drug industry as it relates to birth control.

For example, despite internal discussions about the dangers of asbestos in their talc products, a memo from 1969 showed how the company planned to assure the public there was no danger. When asked what level of Tremolite (asbestos) exposure would be safe in their product, a J&J company doctor warned that the company had already received safety questions expressing "concern over the possibility of adverse effects on the lungs of babies or mothers," and that "it is not inconceivable that we could become involved in litigation." However, another internal memo revealed that J&J trained employees to tell customers that asbestos "has never been and it never will be" in their baby powder.

The company also appeared to dance around the facts when reporting to the FDA. In 1976, as the FDA considered regulations on asbestos levels in talc products, J&J was eager to demonstrate that they could be trusted to self-police. They told the regulator that no asbestos was "detected in any sample" between December 1972 and October 1973. They conveniently omitted three tests between 1972 and 1975, which did report asbestos findings, including one where levels were identified as "rather high."

Finally, J&J took notice of researchers whose studies posed a threat to their bottom line. A team from Mount Sinai Medical Center led by Irving Selikoff noticed a curious rise in the number of deceased patients who had asbestos fibers in their lung tissue. After ruling out work and other environmental exposures, they theorized that talcum powders could be playing a role. They presented their findings to New York City's environmental protection chief in 1971. Later that same year, another doctor from Mount Sinai found a "relatively small" amount of asbestos in Johnson's Baby Powder. Rather than take action to protect the public, J&J placed the doctors on an internal list of "antagonistic personalities" and labeled Selikoff as the leader of an "attack on talc."

J&J maintains that these internal documents have been taken out of context and that their Baby Powder is and always has been safe. In July 2018, the first of what is likely to be many juries disagreed when they awarded $4.69 billion to women who claimed asbestos in the powder caused their ovarian cancer.

CHAPTER 6

Unsafe at Any Dose

Glancing up from the magazine, you notice a woman across the waiting room. Her gaze is fixed somewhere miles beyond the painting you first thought she was admiring. The nervous bounce of her crossed leg draws your attention, and then you realize she's suffering from one of the most common side effects of hormonal birth control - stunned confusion.

Okay, so that's not an official diagnosis, but chances are you know that look. This is not an annoying 'mind fog' kind of confusion. It's more like the head-spinning, I-don't-understand-what-the-heck-is-happening kind. It's similar to the stunned feeling women experienced as they watched the hearings all those years ago, but women today are still seeking answers.

Several women have described this feeling to me. It can carry you along a variety of paths that all lead to the same painful, gut-punched destination. Some examples:

- The young woman experiencing migraines. She read that it could be warning her of a Pill-induced stroke, but she can't understand why the doctor just acted like it was no big deal.

- Another woman told the doctor she didn't feel like herself. The moodiness and anxiety have become unbearable. Rather than addressing what caused her symptoms and stopping The Pill, the doctor wrote a new prescription... for Prozac.

- Or the woman who, after taking The Pill for over a decade is being tested for an endocrine ailment she didn't even know existed. Making matters worse, her doctor reacted with anger when she asked if it could be related to her years on The Pill.

Facing a chronic or life-threatening disease is bad enough, but the queasiness is amplified when you suddenly question the person you've entrusted with your health.

Most of us consider the doctor-patient relationship sacred. We relinquish a bit of our own free will, trusting the doctor to weigh the benefits versus the risks for us. We take comfort knowing he/she has pledged to 'First do no harm,' not realizing that many doctors no longer take the Hippocratic Oath. Of course, this doesn't mean doctors are intentionally harming patients, but it does point to a systemic divide between the level of trust we place in physicians and their subsequent lack of accountability.

How is it that we can see The Pill linked to so many deaths and chronic diseases, yet doctors still act as if it should come in a Pez dispenser? Where does the cognitive end and the dissonance begin?

The DES Debacle: Origins of Obstinance

To understand where we are and how we got here, it's helpful to study the journey that gave us The Pill.

By 1970, the current dogma that 'The Pill is safe' was well-rooted in the broader medical community. However, after leading physicians expressed their concerns in the first round of hearings and caused great anxiety among women taking birth control, Pill proponents demanded that more 'pro-pill' doctors be included in the hearings.

Sen. Nelson took umbrage with their complaints, noting that all but one of the previous doctors had actually been 'pro-pill,' but all had reservations about its complications and the lack of adequate safety testing. Nonetheless, many of the doctors in the second round of hearings seemed more decidedly biased in favor of The Pill, including Dr. Kenneth Ryan, who stated:

> "I know of no information that indicates that biological properties of the estrogens used in the contraceptive pill are any different than stilbesterol for which we have at least 30 years of clinical experience..." (NPH, Page 6541)

Very reassuring... Unless you were actually familiar with the 30-year history of stilbesterol, also known as diethylstilbestrol (DES). Sir Charles Dodds discovered DES in 1938 and rushed it to market in the public domain. Barbara Seaman explained in her fantastic book, *The Greatest Experiment Ever Performed on Women*, that the English doctor bypassed the patent process hoping it would discourage the Germans from further tests on women prisoners. The Nazis were testing ethinyl estradiol (The same chemical still being used in hormonal birth control) as a chemical sterilization agent in their Auschwitz concentration camp.

Despite his noble intentions, Dodds soon regretted the decision. Without a patent, drug companies around the globe were free to produce DES. He never expected that synthetic hormones would be given to healthy women and was horrified that doctors were prescribing it as hormone therapy for natural menopause.

You Can't Put the Hormones Back in the Tube

Even worse, Dodds soon learned that an American doctor named Karnaky had begun blazing a new trail - doling out DES off-label to 'prevent miscarriages.' Alarmed by the news, Dodds sent Karnaky a study he had personally performed, which showed that the drug actually caused miscarriages in animal subjects. It didn't deter Dr. Karnaky or the many doctors who followed his lead.

Dodds began to feel like he was fighting a monster of his own creation. He was most concerned about how his discovery could affect certain cancers. He sent DES samples to the newly formed National Cancer Institute in the United States, urging them to conduct tests and notify doctors of the potential dangers.

Dodds wasn't alone. The Council on Pharmacy and Chemistry warned that the potential harm of these drugs must be recognized and that there use by physicians "should not be undertaken until further studies have led to a better understanding of the functions of the drug. "

The concerns sent murmurs through the medical community, and many doctors began experimenting with lower doses of DES. By 1940, the editors of the Journal of the American Medical Association (JAMA) felt compelled to add their own warning:

> "It would be unwise to consider that there is safety in using small doses of estrogens, since it is quite possible that the same harm may be obtained through the use of small doses of estrogen if they are maintained over a long period." (JAMA, April 20, 1940)

In 1959, the FDA determined the link to side effects (including male breast growth) was sufficient to ban poultry farmers from using DES as a growth hormone. However, the widespread use of DES in women continued. In fact, it had become standard medical practice by the time Dr. Ryan assured Sen. Nelson's committee that The Pill was just as safe as DES -- an alarming example of how medical dogma often trumps scientific evidence.

Unfortunately, the greater irony of Dr. Ryan's statement didn't materialize until one year after his testimony, when researchers first linked a rare vaginal cancer to the daughters of women who received DES during pregnancy. The FDA reacted by finally listing pregnancy as a contraindication for DES, meaning doctors should stop this practice.

Consumer Groups Take the Lead

You would expect this to be the beginning of the end for DES. Shockingly, the medical community responded with indifference, continuing to prescribe DES for a variety of 'off-label' uses, including: as a morning-after pill, to catalyze the onset of puberty, and the old-faithful - hormone replacement therapy.

It took nearly a decade of passionate effort from consumer movements like DES Action to convince doctors to (mostly) abandon DES. Dozens of lawsuits were filed - some were settled, and some are still pending. And today, there is evidence that the harmful consequences could be affecting a third generation of DES victims.

The current Director of Epidemiology and Biostatistics at the National Cancer Institute, Robert Hoover, M.D. oversees the DES Follow-Up Study to track ongoing repercussions. With identifiable problems now affecting the grandchildren of women who took DES, the disaster hasn't yet moved into the past tense of our nation's history. Despite that, Dr. Hoover says that whenever he gives his general epidemiology lecture, nobody has ever heard of DES. He adds, "There's essentially a whole generation of medical students who don't know the story. The story has such powerful lessons that I think that's a tragedy."

Sidney Wolfe, M.D., who headed up Ralph Nader's Health Research Group, offered this perspective:

"DES is an excellent example of how drug companies behave, how they take advantage of the ways doctors act, and how they make millions of dollars by ignoring evidence of a drug's harmfulness, by failing to get evidence that it is effective, and then by marketing a product that plays on fears and misconception."

Twenty short years after the American Medical Association issued their warning that even small doses of synthetic estrogens were unsafe, their position reversed as they embraced the release of insufficiently tested birth control for millions of women. That is a massive sea change in a short amount of time with no apparent science to support it.

Let the Spin Begin

While the term 'Spin Doctor' wouldn't be coined until much later, it became obvious as the hearings proceeded that some prominent physicians were willing to twist statistics, incorporate doublespeak, and create confusion in any way they could to defend The Pill. They were Spin Doctors in the truest sense. Fortunately, within the context of Senate Hearings, their 'spin' was usually challenged.

Dr. Robert Kistner from Harvard couldn't find a bad thing to say about The Pill if his daughter's life depended on it. However, simple challenges to his testimony made some of his statements seem almost comical. Consider this exchange with Ben Gordon. In an attempt to minimize the British study, he compared Pill deaths to those caused by cigarettes:

In the Name of The Pill

Dr. Kistner: For every pill-induced death in Britain there are at least 1,500 cigarette induced deaths; based on the total sales of the two products during 1967 one cigarette is three time as dangerous to life as one pill.

Mr. Gordon: Dr. Kistner, may I interrupt for just one moment? Since you compared the risks of smoking with that of the pill, do you know of any cases where smoking three packages of cigarettes has caused either serious illness or death? Three packages?

Dr. Kistner: Smoking three packages?

Mr. Gordon: Right.

Dr. Kistner: Obviously the answer to that question is no.

Mr. Gordon: I have here the proceedings of a conference held... at the headquarters of the American Medical Association... there are case reports, several reports where people have either died or have become seriously injured taking the pill for only 3 months, in other words, three packages of pills.

Dr. Kistner: Is there a cause and effect relationship demonstrated or proved?

Mr. Gordon: Well, it just says "Case reports: Thrombosis and embolism in patients taking the pill."

Dr. Kistner: There is no cause and effect relationship so far as I can understand.

Mr. Gordon: They said the same thing about tobacco.

Then, there was this exchange with Senator McIntyre after Dr. Kistner suggested he didn't think doctors should be burdened with telling women about every side effect associated with The Pill:

Sen. McIntyre: ...Could you distinguish for me the difference between a side effect and a complication?

Dr. Kistner: Yes. A side effect of a drug is one that is generally accepted as occurring in some individuals as an undesirable effect other than that for which the drug is given. If one takes estrogen, one frequently becomes nauseated, estrogen "pulls in" sodium and some women don't excrete the excess fluid and they become edematous and "blow up." These are side effects: but if a woman takes estrogen and gets a blood clot and dies that is a complication.

Sen. McIntyre: That is more than a complication.

[Laughter]

Today, the spin is just as silly, but the humor is missing. No longer are the distortions challenged. What used to be a laughable punch line is now presented as a valid counterpoint.

Strokes Linked to The Pill

In 2012, the *New England Journal of Medicine* published the results of an extensive Danish study showing that women on birth control pills or other hormonal contraceptives are up to twice as likely to have a stroke or heart attack than non-users, but a funny thing happened to the story on its way to the press. Industry experts analyzed, mitigated, and diluted it beyond recognition.

ABC News offered the most balanced report. Their story begins with a young woman, a 'former smoker and birth control pill user' who suffered a stroke. However, after sharing some of the details of the study, they downplayed the results with the aid of a Spin Doctor, a gynecologist, to be exact, who said, "...pregnancy is far more likely to cause an MI or stroke than hormonal contraception."

An off-handed dismissal like this has no place in a serious news story unless the person responding can cite their sources.

Don't Question The Pill

One could argue that it's good journalism to seek out a dissenting voice – to effectively present both sides of the story. In this case, I disagree. It's dangerous. The journalist gives the impression that the biased opinion of a pill proponent is equivalent to the scientific findings of a comprehensive 15-year, peer-reviewed study.

I have to admit reading the responses from 'expert' physicians frequently brings out my snarky side. Consider the dissenting voices from these Spin Doctors in articles related to the same Danish study.

Huffington Post interviewed Dr. Diana Petitti, who told them, "The amount of attention paid to these minuscule risks...detracts attention from more salient issues, like preventing unwanted pregnancy." Minuscule risks?! I'm not sure, but I think Dr. Petitti is saying she would rather double her daughter's chance of having a stroke than risk her getting pregnant.

Later in the same article, Dr. Kathy Hoeger explained, "The risk might be as much as two times, but when you know that the rates are 1 in 10,000, you're just bringing it up to 2 to 4 in 10,000." Those numbers sound so cute, but when you think about a conservative estimate of 13 million women in the US currently on hormonal contraception - we could be subjecting an <u>*additional*</u> 3,900 women per year to strokes and heart attacks.

My favorite may be Dr. Isaac Schiff, who told Boston.com, "I would say in many ways, this is a good news story. This is a lengthy, large study that helps to confirm that the birth control pill is relatively safe, recognizing that no drug is 100 percent safe." He's ecstatic that The Pill *only* doubles the risk! He probably turned summersaults when he read that women on The Pill also have a 35 percent higher risk of developing multiple sclerosis, a 50 percent higher risk of developing lupus, and could triple their chances of having Crohn's Disease!

Dissenting Voices

So, why is it dangerous to present these dissenting voices? Imagine you're a young woman who's just been diagnosed with a chronic disease. You begin puzzling the pieces together and recall that your first symptoms appeared within weeks or months of starting The Pill. You take your suspicions to Google, and stumble upon an article that confirms your fears... or does it?

So, you click on another article. For example, the lupus article mentioned above, and read, "The risk was greatest during the first three months after starting 'the

Pill' -- when there was a 2.5-fold increased risk." You think you're onto something, but then a world-renowned physician is quoted as saying, "One shouldn't oversell this. Women taking oral contraceptives need to weigh the risk/benefit of unexpected pregnancy versus a very small increase in lupus." We can't blame the reader for concluding her diagnosis probably didn't have to do with The Pill after all.

Forgotten Prophet

As Dr. Hugh Davis' told us in his opening testimony at the hearings, "No one, as the FDA report was careful to point out, has the slightest idea what long-range effects may result from such chronic use of the pill for 15, 20, or even 30 years."

Discussing the many known metabolic side effects that accompany The Pill, *The Lancet* had offered this warning the previous October, "These changes are unnecessary for contraception and their ultimate effect on the health of the user is unknown. But clearly, they cannot be ignored, since they raise the possibility of irreversible structural changes, such as arteriosclerosis, after 10 or 20 years. In view of these doubts, the wisdom of administering such compounds to healthy women for many years must be seriously questioned."

They may have been unsure of exactly what the long-term effects would be, but the pages of the hearings are filled with statements proven prophetic by fifty years of hindsight. Many of the raised concerns have become reality, with the redefinition of strokes skewed toward younger victims being just one example.

When you read the hearing transcripts, the feeling of trepidation leaps from the pages. Witness after witness expresses varying degrees of discomfort with either The Pill or the process by which it was approved. One can't help but wonder, with so many questions, concerns, and doubts, why was The Pill ever approved? And why, for God's sake, was it allowed to stay on the market? Well, the hearings actually provided an unsettling answer for those questions too.

CHAPTER 7

A Greater Social Concern

In an address to the Association of American Medical Colleges in 1969, the year before the hearings, the Nobel Prize winner, Dr. Frederick Robbins articulated thoughts on a new paradigm for healthcare:

> "The dangers of overpopulation are so great that we may have to use certain techniques of conception control that may entail considerable risk to the individual woman."

This statement sent a wave of gasps across the audience of medical school deans, but less than a year later, the hearings would prove that Dr. Robbins was no rogue outlier. Overpopulation was already a hot-button issue, but most people saw it as a third-world problem. Dr. Robbins' statement demonstrated that the population-control movement was actually hitting much closer to home. He may have been among the first to express it so publicly, but the hearings would reveal that thought leaders throughout the medical and political realms had been actively engaged in making his ideal a reality for quite some time.

It is important for us to grasp how seriously entrenched this ideology was among the business and political leaders of that time so we can understand how it influenced their decision-making, and how those decisions still have an impact on us today.

The Population Bomb

Population concerns exploded onto the scene a year earlier when Paul Ehrlich's massively popular book, *The Population Bomb*, hit bookstores everywhere. Mr. Ehrlich wrote the book after his family took an unsettling trip to Delhi, India. He filled its pages with sensational predictions about the catastrophic effects of global overpopulation:

"A *minimum* of ten million people, most of them children, will starve to death each year of the 1970s. But this is a mere handful compared to the numbers that will be starving before the end of the century. And it is now too late to take action to save many of those people."

Mr. Erhlich's doomsday forecasts coupled with almost nightly dire predictions on network newscasts left the nation panicked about overpopulation. After the world's population topped 3.5 billion, Walter Cronkite reported, "Net world population is increasing by 23 people every ten seconds. It's clear that world population growth remains completely out of control."

As more and more people bought into the movement's cries for Zero Population Growth, leaders like Erhlich and Robbins felt comfortable to reveal their bold plans for coercive tactics intended to curb population growth. Speaking at the US national conference for UNESCO in 1969, Mr. Erhlich proposed adding sterility drugs to the nation's food supply and water reservoirs.

Although the idea of tainting food and water supplies never really caught on, the bold rhetoric continued boiling behind the scenes. As it became clear the general public was never going to embrace their most outrageous desires, population control enthusiasts began to speak in more palatable terms. Occasionally, however, one of them would speak a little too frankly to the press, and it would cause a stir. Just months before the Nelson Pill Hearings took place, President Nixon established a separate Office of Population within USAID and gave them a $50 million budget. In 1977, the Director of this Population Program, Dr. Ray Ravenholt, may have been a little too transparent when he told the St. Louis Post Dispatch that his agency's goal was to sterilize twenty-five percent of the women on the planet.

Population Politics

Politically speaking, the population-control movement first saw the light of day with the formation of the Draper Committee in the 1950s. After previously serving on Eisenhower's staff during World War II, General William Draper formed this influential committee, which recommended population-control programs be tied to military assistance in countries struggling with poverty issues.

Government sponsored population control sounded menacing, and the civilian population didn't react well to the Draper Report. President Eisenhower ultimately rejected the report, contending that population problems in other countries were not a concern of the United States government.

However, his hedging seemed to be more a matter of political expediency. Once out of office, he joined another former president, Harry S. Truman as honorary co-chairs of the Planned Parenthood Federation. Though the term "population control" was still being rejected by the public-at-large, the movement suddenly had colossal political clout.

This was a fascinating time for the population control movement. The political elite from both parties in the US seemed to be fully on-board with the need to limit population growth. However, because the idea so repulsed the average voter, the politicians were caught in a delicate balancing act. US voters weren't the only ones listening to their population control arguments incredulously. In 1965, at the Second World Population Conference in Belgrade, the American representative, Frank Lorimer stated, "We have 200 million people now, we will have 300 million by 1980. Wouldn't we be better off with 100 million people less?" To which, the Russian delegate responded, "What is the matter with you Americans, don't you like people?"

The population control movement knew they had a problem with optics, but they were also smart enough to know that cunning manipulation of the language could pave the way for the social engineering they desired. So, they tweaked their pitch to focus on individual responsibility. Their new rally cry centered on family planning and birth control rather than population control, and within a decade, they managed to get birth control legalized and The Pill approved by the FDA.

As a side note, when Dr. Alan Guttmacher, the president of the Planned Parenthood Federation, sought to strengthen ties in minority communities, he approached the National Negro Advisory Council previously established by the Birth Control Federation of America. It was Malcolm X who suggested that 'family planning' would be more palatable than 'birth control.' According to notes taken at that meeting, "His reason for this was that people, particularly Negroes, would be more willing to plan than to be controlled."

Lyndon B. Johnson became the first sitting President to speak publicly in favor of population control. The year was 1965. At a speech celebrating the 20th anniversary of the United Nations, Johnson called upon all member nations to "wage together an international war on poverty." He pleaded with them to protect our fragile heritage, offering this food for thought:

> "Let us in all our lands--including this land--face forthrightly the multiplying problems of our multiplying populations and seek the answers to this most profound challenge to the future of all the world. Let us act on the fact that less than $5 invested in population control is worth $100 invested in economic growth."

Fear Becomes Zeitgeist

By the time the 1968 presidential election rolled around, overpopulation fears had woven their way into the national zeitgeist. Still, the concerns regarding unsustainable population growth were mainly seen as a foreign problem, not a domestic one. The Republican Party's Foreign Policy platform leading up to the elections offered this perspective:

> "The world-wide population explosion in particular, with its attendant grave problems, looms as a menace to all mankind and will have our priority attention. In all such areas we pledge to expand and strengthen international cooperation."

President Richard Nixon stayed true to the promise. It would eventually become evident that 'cooperation' actually meant 'coercion.' Within months of taking office, Nixon delivered a Special Message to Congress on the Problems of Population Growth. Declaring that 'population growth is among the most important issues we face,' he called for 'expanded action and greater coordination' of international population control programs through the United Nations.

He also announced his plans to establish a commission that would evaluate the state of population growth. He appointed John D. Rockefeller to oversee the task. The commission's subsequent report wasted no time in summing up their findings. The first paragraph offered this perspective, "After two years of concentrated effort, we have concluded that, in the long run, no substantial benefits will result from further growth of the Nation's population."

In the Name of The Pill

The Draper Report may have been a failure initially, but by the time General Draper testified at the Nelson Pill Hearings, he proudly dropped the names of some of the influential leaders who had thrown their support behind population control – the Presidents - Nixon, Eisenhower, Johnson, and even Kennedy 'authorized our Government for the first time to help other nations achieve population limitation.'

He explained how they had worked through the United Nations, using the World Health Organization, UNICEF, and the World Bank to provide aid to countries and leaders who would 'promote' population limitation in their countries.

General Draper also offered some insight into the work being done at home. He praised Senator Joseph Tydings and the young Representative George H.W. Bush for their work on a bill that 'will greatly speed up our own domestic family planning programs.' Interestingly, he also mentioned the work of a couple of unelected officials - Dr. Louis Hellman from the FDA, and a young counsel to the President named Rumsfeld. He emphatically declared, "Mr. Donald Rumsfeld [is] loyally devoted to carrying out President Nixon's 5-year program [to reduce population growth]."

There can be no argument that a mighty group of powerful men and women were hell-bent on curbing population growth, and they weren't about to let safety concerns surrounding The Pill get in their way. Or, as General Draper put it, "The decade of the sixties has been the decade of comprehension. The decade of the seventies must become the decade of all-out action."

The Hearings Turn Orwellian

With a new decade upon them, the anti-population evangelists prepared to kick into high gear. And, their misguided enthusiasm spawned some memorable Orwellian moments at the Pill Hearings.

One of the enduring concepts from Orwell's classic, *1984*, is 'Doublethink,' which the author described this way:

> "To know and not to know, to be conscious of complete truthfulness while telling carefully constructed lies, to hold simultaneously two opinions which cancel out, knowing them to be contradictory and believing in both of them, to use logic against logic, to repudiate morality while laying claim to it...consciously to induce unconsciousness, and then, once again, to become unconscious of the act of hypnosis you had just performed."

Perhaps the greatest example of this brand of cognitive dissonance came early in the hearings from the testimony of Dr. Roy Hertz. He had been the Chairman of the task force addressing cancer for the FDA Advisory Committee looking into the safety of The Pill (prior to the hearings). The Chairmen of the various task forces along with Dr. Louis Hellman, who was overseeing all the task forces, unanimously agreed that The Pill was "safe within the intent of the legislation" (more on that in a moment). Dr. Hertz's testimony provided detailed evidence, which heavily suggested: "oral contraceptives would tend to heighten the body's natural propensity toward cancer."

In the Name of The Pill

After demonstrating that, early researchers feared the effect these potent chemicals might have on cancer, he explained that their studies had been limited because of the urgency to get these new agents on the market. He said the worldwide enthusiasm for The Pill had "hampered a truly comprehensive and objective evaluation of its merits and demerits."

Admitting that population pressures influenced the decision to release questionable drugs to the public was bad enough, but then Dr. Hertz noted that just before the FDA endorsed The Pill, the federal government ordered all poultry producers to stop using synthetic estrogens for fattening chickens because they were known to cause cancer in animals.

Each minute of Dr. Hertz's testimony seemed to be more alarming than the previous, leaving reporters in a frenzy. The madness climaxed with a line that became the next morning's headline in newspapers across the country:

"[Estrogens] are to breast cancer what fertilizer is to the wheat crop."

Seeking clarity, Sen. Nelson interrupted Dr. Hertz frequently, but he confessed to being puzzled when Dr. Hertz said:

"The application of these medications in their present state of knowledge constitutes a highly experimental undertaking. That the individual called upon to take these materials, particularly for prolonged periods of time, should be regarded as, in effect, a volunteer for an experimental undertaking."

Sen. Nelson reminded Dr. Hertz that he and the other Task Force Chairmen, along with Dr. Hellman had unanimously declared The Pill to be safe in their report to the FDA. Yet, they all seemed to be saying something else in the aftermath. He read a quote from Dr. Hellman that appeared in the *Obstetrics and Gynecological News*, "If I were a young lady these days and had any fear of cancer I probably would use an intrauterine device." To which, Sen. Nelson asked, "Is there anybody who isn't concerned about cancer?"

Dr. Hertz refused to comment on any statements taken 'out of context,' but did say that he hadn't agreed with the sentence in the report that proclaimed The Pill to be 'safe within the intent of the legislation.' He explained:

> "This was unanimously approved by the committee in open vote as representing an adequate statement of the consensus of the committee... However, there is no inconsistency here in the sense that this represents the Chairman's Summary."

Doublethink...

In fact, the Task Force's very proclamation that The Pill was "safe within the intent of the legislation" was doublethink. The legislation they were referring to was the Kefauver-Harris Amendment that changed the FDA protocol in the wake of the Thalidomide scandal. The legislation gave the FDA more power, and put more focus on the efficacy of drugs during the approval process. The Task Force twisted the interpretation of this focus on efficacy – contorting it to the point that they were finally able to work the word 'safe' into a sentence about The Pill, which appeared to be Dr. Hellman's singular goal.

How to Treat 'Others'

Dr. Herbert Ratner made it clear in his testimony that not only was he concerned about The Pill's safety, but he was also disturbed by the behavior of some of his colleagues. He reminded his fellow doctors of Plato's Laws (Greek pagination 491), "...where Plato distinguishes between the physicians who took care of slaves and the one who took care of freemen. Whereas the slave-doctor prescribed 'as if he had exact knowledge' and gave orders 'like a tyrant,' the doctor of freemen went 'into the nature of the disorder,' entered 'into discourse with the patient and his friends' and would not 'prescribe for him until he has first convinced him.'"

Unfortunately, the majority of doctors who testified followed another line of reasoning – 'the ends justified the means.' Their perspective was best summed up in a threatening tone from Dr. John McCain (not to be confused with the former US Senator), "The population explosion is of overwhelming worldwide importance. It threatens the very foundations of national existence. Unless the explosion is moderated, radical methods of population control, rather than family planning, may be required."

Listening to the testimonies, you begin to understand that the same rules didn't apply to all. For example, Dr. McCain explained that the health risks of The Pill were worth it if a woman found herself in an "unplanned pregnancy, [because of] the risks the infant faces, the socio-economic situation..." He continued, "I will be frank in my statements here, that when I am speaking with doctors, I will give a little different interpretation of my opinion regarding the risks of contraceptive pills than when I am speaking to indigent patients."

Dr. Louis Hellman was a little more specific in his testimony (This is the same Dr. Hellman who chaired the FDA Advisory Committee, and who General Draper described as being fully on-board with President Nixon's five-year population plan). He described a "colored" patient of his from "a ghetto area, she had two children." He fretted that he could no longer give her oral contraceptives because she had a stroke, and he was afraid another child would put her "right back on welfare." Never mind that another stroke might put this mother of two right into the grave. Then again, her health probably wasn't his top priority. As the committee chairman, he said one of The Pill's major benefits was that it "has made the problem of population control immeasurably easier."

Then there was Dr. Joseph Goldzieher, who practiced in San Antonio, Texas. He testified that most of the side effects were "largely inconveniences." Here's how he viewed the difference in patients, "If a woman can really afford another pregnancy, like a doctor's wife, she is the one that is going to complain bitterly about these inconveniences. But poor Mrs. Gonzales who has 10 children, and cannot afford the 11th – she will not complain. She may be afraid that if she does complain, they won't give her the free pills."

By the end of the first round of hearings, Sen. Nelson grew exasperated by the attitude of population-control-at-any-cost. After Dr. McCain lamented that the list of complications was too long to discuss with patients, the senator asked where he stood on informed consent and full disclosure, to which Dr. McCain played a game of semantics, "What is meant by full disclosure? How full does it have to be to be classified as full disclosure?"

Dr. McCain's reply was subtler than some of the previous in regards to differing levels of treatment for women who 'need' family planning, but Sen. Nelson felt compelled to clarify his personal stance on overpopulation and how it factored into medical care. It's a rather long quote, but it's important to digest what the senator was saying:

> "I happen to be very concerned and would endorse the [earlier] statement you made about population. I think the most critical matter facing humankind is the overpopulation of the planet. I have friends who feel that way and think, therefore, you had better not tell anybody about the side effects because one of the benefits of the risk-benefit ratio includes overpopulating the planet. I have never understood that to be the responsibility of the physician, *to make a sacrifice of a patient for the purposes of some wider sociological gain*. But this is the attitude of many people who have talked to me, including many of the doctors that I have talked to. Their position is that *disclosing the concern of the profession and the facts about the pill threatens the cause of birth control* and limitations in population growth. They apparently feel, and some of them have in fact conceded to playing the part of "Big Brother" to all the rest of the women in the world. *They conclude that population*

control is so important that no one should be informed about the pill for fear they will not use it."

Aside from the hearings, 1970 was a busy year for Sen. Nelson because he was also organizing another major event that would go on to become an annual affair. As the founder of Earth Day, Sen. Nelson was a known environmentalist who really did have his own serious concerns about overpopulation – but he clearly drew the line somewhere short of sacrificing humans.

The Population Patrol

The hearings left little doubt that information was being suppressed at every level. While much of the debate centered around informed consent and the individual patient-doctor relationship, it became apparent that dangers swirling around The Pill weren't even being fully disclosed to the physicians themselves. As it turns out, Dr. David Clark's famous quote about The Pill being granted some sort of 'diplomatic immunity' may have been a dramatic understatement.

While it can't be proven that information was intentionally suppressed, Dr. Ratner threw down the gauntlet in his testimony:

"It should be distressing to American physicians that although the pill was first discovered, researched, clinically tested, marketed, and widely used in the United States, and although the number of women using the pill in the United States far exceeds the number in other countries, and although there were four United States-dominated committees appointed to investigate safety, it is not the United States with

its much vaunted scientific resources and superior health accomplishments that resolved the vital question of the association of thromboembolism with the pill.
"It was resolved by England, a medically socialized country whose resources, supposedly, do not compare to ours."

Today, it would still be difficult to prove that information is intentionally being withheld from the public, but there are signs that, at the very least, pertinent information is being downplayed and mitigated. When you begin to research side effects associated with The Pill, you see certain responses that are so ubiquitous they seem to have come from a playbook. Search for a news story on any side effect related to hormonal contraceptives, and you're likely to find at least one of these responses somewhere in the story:

1) **This doesn't prove a connection** – This phrase is usually followed by, "More research needs to be done." It has confounded those with safety concerns since the early days because no benchmark is ever established to say what *would* prove a connection for the naysayers.
2) **This doesn't mean women should stop taking The Pill** – It's amazing how frequently this line comes from the lead investigator who has just uncovered the link to a chronic or deadly complication. It reads almost like a mea culpa to the drug industry.

A Greater Social Concern

3) **This only affects _____ women per 10,000** – Naysayers frequently use statistical acrobatics to reframe the numbers so that they seem less significant. However, with a low-end estimate of 13 million women taking hormonal contraceptives, any number per 10,000 adds up quickly.
4) **The risk is greater if you are over 35 or smoke** - This is usually true, but the sleight-of-hand implies if you are young and don't smoke, you have nothing to worry about - which couldn't be further from the truth.
5) **The benefits still outweigh the risks** – Benefit to whom versus risk to whom?

Many prominent physicians are still willing to perpetuate this pattern of denial and obfuscation whenever a new study is published. The Nelson Pill Hearings and the DES debacle both demonstrated how medical dogma often trumps scientific evidence if the right pressures exist.

At this point, you may be wondering why I'm spending so much ink on social issues, which don't deal directly with the dangers of hormonal contraceptives. In my conversations over the past few years, I've discovered that this is the single biggest hurdle for people to get over when contemplating the 'big picture' ramifications of The Pill. And, quite honestly, it was the hardest thing for me to intellectualize during my research.

Every time I discovered a new, dangerous side effect, my mind would come back to the same thought, "If The Pill really does this, why is it still on the market? If it contributes to all these complications, how can any doctor still say that the benefits outweigh the risks?"

As I read the transcripts of the Nelson Pill Hearings, I understood for the first time the strength of the population control movement. The pages of testimony came alive as I experienced the greatest epiphany in all of my research. I witnessed some of the most influential doctors of that era explaining the dramatic shift in the benefit-to-risk paradigm – the benefit to society versus the risk to the individual patient. They believed they were on a mission to save the planet from unsustainable population growth. In their minds, the end justified the means.

How Low Would They Go?

With the western world's elites united in a fight against population growth, the drug companies were set for a big payday, and they weren't going to let anything stand in their way. The hearings unveiled some of the corruption behind bringing birth control to market, but it would take a couple of decades before many of the industry's more unsavory practices would come to light. Unfortunately, by then, birth control was solidly embedded in the culture.

In 1986, Constance Bailey sued G.D. Searle for damages related to severe liver damage after she began taking their birth control pills. A former FDA official testified that the company had faked results in their drug safety tests, and had removed data demonstrating that test animals developed liver tumors while on the drug. Even the FDA commissioner chimed in that this cast doubt on the believability of all drug safety tests.

A Greater Social Concern

Unfortunately, the dangers of birth control aren't limited to hormonal contraceptives. A.H. Robins Co. was notified as early as 1971 that their Daikon Shield IUD was causing an alarming number of septic abortions. Anticipating a drop in sales, they offered to sell bulk packages of the device to Dr. Ravenholt's USAID office at a 48 percent discount. Nearly a decade later, several thousand users brought a lawsuit against the company for damages. An attorney for Robins testified that he had been ordered to burn potentially incriminating documents in 1975. Judge Miles Lord reprimanded the company's executives with this statement:

> "The only conceivable reasons you have not recalled this product are that it would hurt your balance sheet and alert women who already have been harmed that you may be liable for their injuries.
> You have taken the bottom line as your guiding beacon and the low road as your route. This is corporate irresponsibility at its meanest."

A Mass Population Experiment

In her enlightening book, *Reproductive Rights and Wrongs*, Betsy Hartmann breaks down the fallacy of overpopulation in the Third World and demonstrates how population control policies influenced the current look of birth control here in the US. She writes:

> "Married to population control, family planning has been divorced from the concern for women's health and well-being that inspired the first feminist crusaders for birth control... A family planning program designed to improve health and to expand

women's control over reproduction looks very different indeed from one whose main concern is to reduce birth rates as fast as possible."

She suggests that if a contraceptive policy were genuinely concerned with women's health, it would do more to promote barrier methods that also protect against sexually transmitted diseases or natural methods that allow for child spacing without introducing internal pollutants to the woman's body.

In fact, natural forms of fertility awareness have enjoyed growing popularity among young women in recent years. This shouldn't be confused with the highly ineffective rhythm method. Nor is it exclusive to religious-based 'natural family planning.' While the Creighton Model and Billings Method have begun to appeal to women outside the Roman Catholic faith, there are also successful secular versions of fertility awareness available from various sources.

Planned Parenthood claims that fertility awareness methods are only about 80 percent effective. However, a report published in the *Osteopathic Journal of Medicine* in 2013 found the overall effectiveness of fertility awareness methods when used correctly to be greater than 95 percent (Creighton 99.5%; Billings 97%). These numbers are comparable to The Pill, but without all the risks that good doctors, like Dr. John Laragh tried to warn us about in the Nelson Pill Hearings:

> "The history of powerful drugs simply reveals for us that sometimes, 8 or 10 years go by before a very serious side effect is appreciated... In a drug like the oral contraceptive, we have a very unique situation,

because this is a mass population experiment ... We have never had a medication in which the commitment for its usage might be daily for 20 years... I think we just have to have a great respect for what we are doing..."

Like so many of the warnings issued at the hearings, Dr. Laragh's statement proved prophetic. Many women are taking The Pill daily for 20 years or more, and very serious side effects have appreciated. However, we lost any sense of respect for the grand experiment.

CHAPTER 8

The Dose Makes the Poison

As a result of the hearings, The Pill became the first medication ever required to include an information booklet for patients. Unfortunately, the oft-ignored booklet also meets informed consent requirements, which may explain why so few doctors take the time to warn patients about side effects.

In the aftermath of the hearings, drug manufacturers also rolled out new, lower-dose versions of The Pill, and claimed they were safer than the previous generations. Again, these statements were made without adequate testing, but this time, the claims went unchecked, even as hormonal contraception expanded to include rings, patches, injections, and IUDs. None of them have been proven safe. In fact, Bayer HealthCare Pharmaceuticals, the maker of today's most popular birth control brands, Yaz and Yasmin, paid out $2.04 billion to settle over

10,000 blood-clot lawsuits as of January 2016. They paid another $57 million to heart attack and stroke victims, and $21.5 million for those who suffered gallbladder damage. Those numbers have likely increased, as several thousand cases remain unsettled and more are filed each day.

On the Dole

To the senators who had taken up the cause, the patient information booklet and lower-dose formulations signaled they had accomplished their mission. In fact, when I first contacted Ben Gordon and told him I was researching complications associated with hormonal birth control, he asked me why I was so interested. He said those first generation pills were so different than what women have today, and asked if today's pills weren't much better.

I'll never forget his reaction when I told him about the similar problems associated with today's birth control. His voice grew distant and apprehensive, "It's still happening."

There was a knowing in the way he said it - as if he had expected as much from the drug companies. I felt horrible for having told him - like I'd just punched a 102-year-old man in the stomach. While he lamented the fact that no other politician has 'taken up the torch,' there is another senator who did maintain course throughout the entirety of his long career.

As a young, first-term senator from Kansas, you will recall that Sen. Dole eagerly tore into physicians who suggested The Pill had safety issues. Ironically (or perhaps, fittingly), young people today may be more likely to know Bob Dole as a pharmaceutical spokesperson who suffered from erectile dysfunction, than as a senator or presidential candidate.

Yet, Sen. Dole was a key figure in two of three major paradigm shifts that changed the regulatory landscape to the benefit of drug companies. In 1980, Sen. Dole co-sponsored the Bayh-Dole Act, legislation which enabled academic institutions and researchers to share in profits from patents they helped develop. While the intention may have been good, the legislation essentially made bedfellows of the industry and those who should be its watchdogs. Suddenly, researchers were working closely with drug companies in hopes of a big payday.

In her wonderful book, *The Truth About the Drug Companies: How They Deceive Us and What to Do About It*, Marcia Angell, M.D. writes extensively about the problems with the Bayh-Dole Act, and how it contributed to the second problematic paradigm shift, Big Pharma's influence on medical education. She described their new relationship this way:

"The Reagan years and Bayh-Dole also transformed the ethos of medical schools and teaching hospitals. These nonprofit institutions started to see themselves as "partners" of industry, and they became just as enthusiastic as any entrepreneur about the opportunities to parlay their discoveries into financial gain. Faculty researchers were encouraged to obtain patents on their work (which were assigned to their universities), and they shared in the royalties... One of the results has been a growing pro-industry bias in medical research—exactly where such bias doesn't belong. "

As a former editor of the prestigious *New England Journal of Medicine*, Dr. Angell became keenly aware of the pharmaceutical industry's influence on medical education, and it doesn't end with the medical schools. Her book goes on to explain how the industry moved to virtually lock down control of continuing medical education, which every doctor must receive in order to maintain their license.

Doctors in every field are required to maintain a certain amount of CME credits each year. The courses to obtain these credits are usually held at beautiful resorts in exotic locations and are sponsored by (to be read, 'paid for by') drug companies relevant to their specialty. Track down a copy of Dr. Angell's book if you'd like a more in-depth explanation of how drug companies have turned CME credits into an extension of their marketing efforts.

In a third paradigm shift, the drug companies brought their control of the message full-circle. They established a new wave of consumerism for their products with direct-to-consumer advertising for prescription medications. The FDA Commissioner at the time, Arthur Hayes asked the companies to stop marketing to the public, warning that it would:

"lead patients to pressure physicians to prescribe unnecessary or un-indicated drugs, increase the price of drugs, confuse patients by leading them to believe that some minor difference represents a major therapeutic advance, potentiate the use of brand-name products rather than cheaper, but equivalent generic drugs and foster increased drug taking in an already overmedicated society."

Perhaps that was the goal. If so, it has been incredibly effective. Today, their influence is nearly as insidious and dangerous as the synthetic hormones still being given to young women.

It's a systemic problem, and the average physician isn't to blame. In many ways, they too are victims of the curriculum. They were educated in institutions that enthusiastically became 'partners of industry,' and they receive Continuing Medical Education from influential doctors, who, in turn, receive massive payouts from Big Pharma.

Of course, it is possible that even the influential teaching doctors really are blind to the damage being done by synthetic hormones. As Upton Sinclair once said, "It is difficult to get a man to understand something when his salary depends upon his not understanding it."

CHAPTER 9

The Green Plasma Mystery

A group of doctors turned detectives may have tackled a case that best demonstrates how little things have changed since those early days of The Pill. It was 2008, well after the current generation of hormonal birth control had been introduced.

While in surgery at the University of Pennsylvania, the doctors were taken aback when a unit of plasma "with a striking green color entered [their] operating room." Plasma is normally straw yellow. So the vivid green appearance troubled them. Although the blood bank assured them the plasma was safe, the anesthesiologist refused the unit and sent it back for disposal.

The team shared photos of the plasma unit with thirty other members of their department who responded with similar bewilderment. They began to investigate this mysterious green phenomenon and reported their findings in the journal, *Anesthesiology*:

> "We could find no reports on green plasma in the past 40 years in either the surgical or the anesthesia literature, which perhaps explains the lack of knowledge on the part of today's clinicians. However, we found several articles dating back to the 1960s."

What they found in the studies from decades prior was that researchers had begun to see a wave of green plasma donations coming from young women shortly after the introduction of The Pill. The source of the color was actually a blue precipitate later identified as the copper-carrying protein, ceruloplasmin. The bright green hue resulted from the mixture of plasma's normal yellow color with an overabundance of the blue protein.

In one of the old studies, researchers noted that estrogen increases copper retention and, consequently, elevates ceruloplasmin levels. So, for their research, they identified fifteen donors who had elevated ceruloplasmin levels and checked their histories. Sure enough, all of them were taking oral contraceptives, and all of them had green plasma.

The current-day doctors at Penn must have been perplexed. Decades earlier, doctors had identified the source of the green color, linked it to oral contraceptives, and then... they just dropped it.

Lots of Loose Ends

While studies related to green plasma may have come to a sudden stop, the effect of synthetic estrogen on copper levels in young birth control patients didn't. In recent years, there has been a lot of discussion about the impact of copper overload or copper toxicity. As a result, scientists have concentrated more on the biological roles of copper and ceruloplasmin.

While it exists as the primary transport vehicle for copper throughout the body, the main function of ceruloplasmin appears to be iron oxidation. However, depending on its surroundings, it can serve as an oxidant or an antioxidant. This means it can take on very different roles depending on where it is in the body and what stew of lipids and proteins surround it.

Subsequent research has demonstrated correlations between copper/ceruloplasmin levels and a whole host of maladies that have also been linked to hormonal birth control. You will read about many of these in Part Two. They include anxiety, depression, infertility, hair loss, headaches, diabetes, high and low blood pressure, and breast cancer. Clinical trials have even demonstrated that therapeutic copper depletion can help stop the spread of breast cancer.

Other studies have shown ceruloplasmin levels to be an effective biomarker for thyroid disease and cancer, as well as heart failure. There seems to be an almost endless parallel between the effects of copper overload and the known side effects of birth control, which isn't surprising since we know an increase in estrogens spawns greater copper retention.

Further studies have also demonstrated that high copper levels can be passed through the placenta. In fact, elevated copper levels in newborns are quite common today. This is significant because high copper levels at birth have been linked to autism, ADHD, and even endometriosis.

Clearly, ceruloplasmin drew the attention of many curious investigators across the medical spectrum over the years. A multitude of published studies have explored the correlation between ceruloplasmin and all these ill effects on the human body, yet the doctors at Penn couldn't find a single piece of literature since 1969 tying it back to birth control or the young women with green plasma.

Hidden Threats to Non-Users

In medical research, it's relatively common to have more questions than answers. However, when hormonal contraceptives are involved, the question-to-answer ratio becomes absurd. It's as if those who control the funding don't want to find many of the answers.

If the final two questions in her letter to Sen. Nelson are any indication, Barbara Seaman must have had the same suspicion. This was her last question, "Why have important investigators found their funds cut off?" I doubt it was coincidental that the preceding question went like this:

> "What hidden threats to the health of non-users are contained in the pill? I am enclosing [clippings] about the green-tinted blood plasma in pill users. Nobody knows what this means, and yet Stanford has apparently decided to go ahead and use such plasma for transfusions anyway."

Incidentally, Ms. Seaman's letter was penned in 1969, the same year as the final 'green plasma' study.

The Green Plasma Mystery

But, halting green plasma studies doesn't make green plasma go away. If it was so common among birth control users, how come so few doctors today have ever seen it? The simple answer is that blood banks did ultimately decide to remove green plasma from their supplies. The American Red Cross came up with visual guidelines for blood components that have been adopted by several other blood services and blood banks around the world.

Ironically, at least one team of modern-day researchers suggests green plasma should "be actively reintroduced into the medical community for transfusion of critically injured and bleeding patients." They argue that, in cases where the patient experiences life-threatening bleeding, green plasma is perfect because of its "superior hemostatic properties" – in other words, its tremendous ability to clot.

If this were an audiobook, this is where I would insert a loud record scratch followed by a dramatic pause to make sure the listener knows we just went off the rails.

Imagine this. Researchers compared green plasma with normal yellow plasma and discovered that the green-tinted samples had higher hypercoagulation values (clotting ability) across the board. Given this knowledge, you might think they would recommend that women with green plasma should be warned about the possibility of clotting disorders, or at the very least, that more tests should be done to see if women with green plasma experience more blood clots. Instead, they saw it as an opportunity to use the Super-Clotting plasma as a resource in the operating room.

Rejecting Women's Plasma

Unfortunately, this callous attitude toward women's health seems to be a continuation of the norm from the early days of The Pill. Indeed, the case of the green plasma mystery offers more damning evidence to affirm Betsy Hartmann's statement that "family planning has been divorced from the concern for women's health and well-being."

While there was much concern about green plasma because of its appearance, something bigger was happening in the realm of the unseen, and it may not be limited to those with green plasma.

Plasma is one of the components derived from donated blood after it has been separated, and a disturbing number of patients were having severe reactions to their plasma transfusions. In 1992, doctors documented the first known fatality related to what is now known as transfusion-related acute lung injury (TRALI). In most cases, their blood pressure would drop, they developed shortness of breath, and their lungs began to fill with fluid. TRALI is essentially an immune response – the recipient's body defending itself against something contained in the donor's blood.

To this day, doctors understand very little about the exact causes of TRALI, but one of the things they were able to confirm early on was that the problem seemed to be tied to female donors. The industry needed to take action as the number of TRALI cases began to climb. It would soon become the leading cause of transfusion-related death.

In 2003, the United Kingdom led the response by implementing a male-predominant policy for plasma donations. The blood-banking industry in the United States followed their lead, and by 2007, recommended that no plasma from female donors be used in transfusions. That's right – for over a decade, the blood-banking industry has avoided using women's plasma for transfusions. When this decision was made, they didn't want a lot of publicity because they were afraid women would stop donating blood altogether.

Their primary hypothesis at the time was that the lung injuries had to do with antibodies contained within the blood of the female donors. Antibodies are proteins produced by the immune system to fight off unrecognized threats such as viruses or bacteria, but researchers pointed out that a woman's body can also create antibodies in reaction to the presence of the father's cells when she becomes pregnant.

The media picked up this convenient storyline and ran with it. At least one major headline proclaimed, "Blood transfusions from women who have been pregnant could kill men." However, it wasn't just men being killed by TRALI, nor were results conclusive that pregnancy-related antibodies were the sole offenders.

We've Got Our Answer

Let's look at another way, specific to women, that antibodies are developed. As far back as 1969, studies revealed that many women on The Pill experienced increased serum levels of certain antibodies. One trial, which focused on the autoimmune disease, lupus, tested women who developed rheumatic symptoms after starting The Pill and found that serum antinuclear antibodies (ANA) were present in a vast majority of these young women. For most of the patients, the abnormalities disappeared when they stopped taking birth control. Today, the ANA blood test is a primary tool used by physicians to assess whether a patient may have systemic lupus erythematosus (SLE).

Antibodies are not unique to lupus. In fact, 'direct evidence of disease-causing antibodies' is the first criterion for a disease to be classified as autoimmune. Anytime the immune system is activated, antibodies will be involved. Consequently, elevated levels of particular antibodies accompany every autoimmune disease.

So, here's where we are in the story arc:

1) Autoimmune Disease is a classification of disease in which nearly 80 percent of all diagnoses are women.

2) TRALI is a severe alloimmune response in transfusion patients, which seems most likely to occur when the donor is a woman. ('Auto' means 'self' so autoimmune is an immune response to antigens from one's self. And, 'allo' means 'other' so this is a response to antigens from outside one's self.)

3) Aside from TRALI, blood banks already had a policy of discarding many plasma donations from young women on birth control because of its unusual appearance, knowing the green hue is caused by a metabolic effect on serum proteins.

4) Hormonal birth control use has been shown to increase the risk of several common autoimmune diseases.

When you add these facts together, you would expect some curious investigator might be eager to see what the correlation is between TRALI-related donors and contraceptive use, yet not a single study exists. To be fair, blood banks exclude people with autoimmune diseases from donating. So, most researchers may assume that risk has already been eliminated. However, several studies, including the lupus study previously mentioned, have shown that these elevated antibody levels can flourish in women on hormonal contraceptives even when they don't display any symptoms and/or before they've been diagnosed with an autoimmune disease.

Never Too Late

Fortunately, blood banks keep detailed records of their donors. After the doctors at Penn put on their sleuth hats and followed the trail of the Green Plasma Mystery, they contacted the blood bank to see if they could obtain ceruloplasmin levels for the returned unit. Unfortunately, it had already been discarded, but the blood bank was able to confirm that the donor was a healthy 27-year-old female graduate student "absent all medical conditions and medications, except for a 5-year history of oral contraceptive use."

Remember, this was 2008, just after US blood banks announced their plans to avoid female plasma as much as possible. While the media was reporting that the issue was only with women who had ever conceived, the sleuth-doctors provided a clue of their own that concern extended beyond just women who had ever been pregnant. They wrote, "Blood banks will not be able to exclude pregnant women or women on birth control pills altogether as plasma donors because they simply will not be able to meet the needs of the country."

The data still exists that could prove whether or not there is a strong association between TRALI and donors who were on contraceptives. It's a question that needs an answer, but I suspect funding will be hard to find.

PART II
The Effect

The second part of this book highlights the many ways women's health has suffered in the wake of decades of hormonal birth control. Some readers will be surprised to learn that the consequences don't just affect women who have taken The Pill. The impact runs much deeper.

I attempted to include the most essential information about each disease even if that means repeating some things from other chapters. I have attempted to treat each chapter as an autonomous essay for the readers who may only want to read about that particular disease. Although, you may find it valuable to read the remainder of Part Two to see the relationship that exists between many of these diseases.

Part Two begins with the original threats, the consequences that even staunch Pill proponents were forced to recognize as side effects from the beginning: Blood Clots, Strokes, Migraines, Heart Disease, Cancer, Sterility, and Psychological Disorders.

The subsequent chapters focus on some side effects that were less recognized in the early days of The Pill. However, today, these may have grown into the gravest threat for women taking hormones. Autoimmune disease wasn't yet a household word when the Nelson Pill Hearings took place. However, some of the doctors' testimonies did focus on individual autoimmune diseases, such as lupus and diabetes. They also discussed certain thyroid and digestive disorders that we now associate with autoimmunity.

Finally, we look at how these potent chemicals threaten life beyond the women taking them every day, and examine potential solutions to change the course of these deadly consequences.

These later chapters focus on the role of hormonal contraceptives as endocrine disruptors. The singular focus on hormonal contraceptives in this book isn't meant to suggest that they are the only chemicals disrupting our endocrine systems. Other chemicals work their way into our systems and mimic natural estrogen. However, media coverage of chemicals disrupting our endocrine systems focuses a disproportionate amount of attention on chemicals like Dioxins, BPA, DDT, even soy. Amazingly, hormonal birth control is rarely even mentioned in these stories.

As we will see, many of these diseases have witnessed a widening gender gap since the introduction of The Pill – meaning more women than men are affected by the disease than was the case before birth control was introduced. This fact alone is enough to incriminate The Pill as a leading suspect, since none of the other endocrine disruptors work in such a sex-specific manner. To omit birth control in any serious conversation on the topic of endocrine disruption is akin to writing a story on major US cities and leaving out New York *and* Los Angeles. The goal of this book is to balance that discussion by placing attention where it belongs – on the most prevalent, potent, and pernicious endocrine disruptor on the planet.

In the Name of The Pill

CHAPTER 10

Migraines:
A Neglected Stop Sign

No sooner had we landed than my phone began to convulse with a cacophony of bells and chimes. Most of the notifications were last minute details about the live broadcast that brought me to town. One voice message was from a coworker letting me know that the producer had canceled our pre-production dinner meeting because she had migraines. He added, "When she eats certain breads, it triggers her headaches."

This happened early in my research on hormonal contraceptives, but I had read enough to know that birth control could cause migraines, and women with migraines were at a higher risk for strokes. I also knew that doctors at the Nelson Pill Hearings testified that birth control pills affect the way a woman's body metabolizes carbohydrates in myriad ways. I had no idea what the mechanism of action could be, but at that moment I would have bet my children's milk money that our producer was on The Pill, and I intended to ask her about it.

This was my client's client. I wondered if it was safe to broach the subject of birth control with her, but I knew the answer before I could even fully form the question in my head. I wouldn't be able to forgive myself if she ever had a stroke, and I hadn't warned her.

The next morning she felt better and was at work for the load-in. When no one else was around, I asked some questions about her headaches, ending with, "I'm curious, did you start getting migraines after you began birth control?"

When you ask a question like that, you know there's a better than zero chance the reaction could be negative. Thankfully, not even a glimmer of disapproval flashed in her eyes as she replied, "Oh no, I took The Pill for a long time before I had my first migraine."

I half-jokingly said, "That's still *after* you started."

We laughed it off, but after sleeping on it, she approached me the next morning, "You know, you may be onto something. I hadn't thought about it, but my migraines did get a lot worse when I switched birth control brands."

Connect the Dots

The correlation between birth control and migraines has been known for decades, as has their connection to an increased risk of stroke. However, two hurdles probably play a key role in preventing patients and their physicians from making the connection in the real world today – those being familiarity and latency.

Migraines

Many side effects of The Pill occur as extremely common ailments, such as breast cancer, strokes, and migraines. Not coincidentally, ailments like migraines have grown even more common in direct correlation to the introduction and prevalence of hormonal contraceptives. Paradoxically, they've become so familiar, so unremarkable that doctors seem to have forgotten about looking for what could be causing the migraines. Essentially, they can't see the tree for the forest.

Some side effects, such as migraines or depression, can happen almost instantaneously. (Even so, doctors frequently miss the connection.) However, it usually takes some time for the symptoms to precipitate. This latency can hinder even the most astute physician from considering hormonal contraceptives as the likely cause of problems. I'm being generous in my phrasing because I can't help but wonder what role fear of litigation might also play in this 'blindness.'

Ultimately, *why* the correlation to birth control is overlooked is less important than the consequences it creates, which include dramatic underreporting of complications. In 1970 while discussing strokes at the Nelson Pill Hearings, Sen. Nelson expressed a prescient concern that doctors' tendencies to downplay the side effects might one day lead to them not being attributed to The Pill at all.

Dr. Herbert Ratner added his perspective, "For the first time in medicine's history, the drug industry has placed at our disposal **a powerful, disease-producing chemical** for use in the healthy rather than the sick." [my emphasis] Yet, forty-five years later, we still have no national registry, no way of tracking patients on birth control so that scientists can conduct comprehensive etiological studies that would connect the dots and precisely reveal the consequences of hormonal contraceptives. In fact, our healthcare reporting system is so fractured we can't even put our finger on an accurate estimate of how many women take hormonal birth control. Estimates from trusted sources range from Guttmacher Institute's estimate of 11 million to 18 million from the Journal for Reproductive Medicine.

The Pill, Migraines, and Strokes

The University of Virginia student health services published a document on their website outlining the definitive link between migraines and strokes. Beyond warning that the "increased risk of stroke is amplified by the use of estrogen-containing birth control methods," the doctors who prepared the document boldly state, "it is **strongly recommended** that women with a personal or family history of migraine headaches should select non-estrogen methods of contraception." [Their emphasis]

This information should be part of every 'informed consent' conversation before a doctor writes the first birth control script. Not to mention the many other complications that need to be discussed. This kind of warning should be the norm. Unfortunately, it's the exception.

Strokes Redefined

It took only three generations of users for hormonal contraceptives to redefine our perception of strokes. A young woman starting on The Pill today may not even realize that when her great-grandmother began birth control, strokes were considered an old person's disease. But, strokes aren't just for grandparents anymore. A recent article in the *Washington Post* leads off with this troubling statement:

"In a study released Wednesday in the *Journal of the American Heart Association*, researchers found that between 2000 and 2010, hospitalizations for ischemic stroke, the most common type, dropped nearly 20 percent overall – but among people ages 25 to 44, there was a sharp 44 percent increase in the rate."

There are a couple of other interesting facts later in the article - or rather, one interesting fact, and another made interesting by its glaring omission. The first comes from a description of the study:

"The data analyzed includes information on 8 million hospital stays and came from the Nationwide Inpatient Sample, the largest publicly available database in the United States on these patients."

In stressing the importance of an extensive database, the author underscores the necessity for a national registry to track patients so that important lines can be drawn. Of course, the second part is that the lines actually need to be drawn. Amazingly, the *Post* attributes the rise in strokes among younger adults "to the same lifestyle risk factors traditionally found in older patients, such as obesity, diabetes, and high blood pressure."

It isn't until much later in the article that they include:

"Each year significantly more women die from stroke than from breast cancer — and yet many women think of stroke as a man's disease. According to a 2015 national survey, only 11 percent of the 1000 women surveyed could identify female-specific stroke risk factors, like migraine headaches with aura, hormone-replacement therapy, oral contraception, and pregnancy, particularly in the final month and postpartum."

Maybe women would stand a better chance of identifying these factors if journalists dared include them in the "lifestyle risk factors" mentioned at the beginning of the article.

It may be uncomfortable but if you know a woman who suffers migraines, don't hesitate to ask her if she's on hormonal contraceptives. Then, please share the facts about migraines and birth control.

CHAPTER 11

More Deadly Blood Clots

The science linking birth control pills to strokes hasn't changed. As far as I can tell, no one has disputed the correlation since *The Lancet* first published Dr. Victor Wynn's study in 1966. Ischemic strokes, the type that occurs when a clot temporarily blocks the blood flow to a part of the brain, account for nearly 90 percent of all strokes today.

Unfortunately, the brain isn't the only part of the body susceptible to serious damage from blood clots. Researchers soon discovered a growing percentage of young women on The Pill were also suffering from dangerous, even deadly thromboemboli and pulmonary emboli.

Testimony Without Equivocation

Pay attention to this excerpt from Dr. Alan Guttmacher's testimony at the Nelson Pill Hearings. Dr. Guttmacher was the founding president of Planned Parenthood/World Population, and was arguably the staunchest Pill proponent to ever live:

> "We know the facts about thromboembolism. I think this is pretty uncontested. We know the facts about development of high blood pressure in a certain small proportion of patients. We know the fact that certain patients get depressed on the pill. These are the facts we are all privy to."

Earlier in the hearings, Dr. J. Edwin Wood explained the phenomenon of clotting in healthy young women. He described how the veins in the extremities of women on oral contraceptives begin to dilate. Because these wider veins are carrying the same amount of blood, the blood flow slows down, which leads to relative stagnation. This is called stasis and can contribute to clotting of the blood. The exquisite detail of his testimony reveals that the facts about hormonal contraceptives, strokes, and emboli were well known in 1970, yet all these decades later, they still haven't made it into the medical school curriculum, and the medical industry has done nothing to address these concerns – nor has the pharmaceutical industry.

In fact, the new formulations of hormonal birth control like Yaz, contain drospirenone and have been found to be two to three times *more likely* to cause blood clots than previous generations. The French drug safety agency, ANSM released findings that the new pills were responsible for twice as many deaths as the older formulations.

Never Just a Number

I often search the internet for personal stories of young women who have suffered the devastating consequences of birth control. These stories remind me why I've taken up this fight. They also help me not to be desensitized by statistics. Each new digit is more than a tick of the tally. It represents someone's daughter, a girlfriend, a wife... a young woman who suffered needlessly.

Shortly after a jury awarded Dewayne Johnson $289 million in his lawsuit against Monsanto for damages from using their product, Roundup, it inspired an avalanche of new lawsuits against the company. I wrote about the decision for the website, Hormones Matter, and related it to one of these birth control stories. Here's an excerpt:

> The Roundup avalanche began with one person. At least for a day or two, everyone knew who Dewayne Johnson was. His case focused a lot of attention on the risks of Roundup and the manufacturer's willingness to overlook those dangers for the sake of profits.
>
> There are innumerable heartbreaking stories of young women who have been maimed or killed by their birth control. Any one of these could have been 'the One' that launched an avalanche against hormonal birth control. The internet is filled with these stories. Let's pick one:

In 2011, the Canadian Broadcast Company (CBC) ran a story on a mother who was suing Bayer Healthcare for the death of her daughter. A healthy 18-year old, Miranda Scott went to the gym after 5-weeks on Yasmin. She collapsed while on the elliptical machine unable to breathe. An autopsy revealed she died from pulmonary emboli, blood clots in the lungs. It was only after her death that her mother began researching Yasmin, and discovered it was the likely cause of her blood clots and very early death.

At this point, Bayer had already paid out over $1 billion in blood clot related settlements. But, here's how they responded to the lawsuit in a statement to the CBC:

"We are very disappointed in Justice Crane's decision to certify a class in Ontario in an ongoing lawsuit regarding Yaz and Yasmin. No decision has been made on the merits of the case. We have filed a request with the Court for leave to appeal the decision and are evaluating our legal options... At Bayer patient safety comes first and we fully stand behind, Yaz and Yasmin."

Seven years have passed since Miranda Scott's death, and Bayer has paid out more than another billion dollars in settlements. I understand the real reason why Bayer still stands behind their product – it's a moneymaker, which honestly probably ranks a little higher than patient safety in their eyes. What I can't understand is why women's health advocates still stand behind hormonal birth control.

It Gets Painfully Real

The deaths of these young women is not something that is in our past, nor is it limited to a single product or even a single type of product. Killer blood clots form with every generation of synthetic hormones - from pills, injections, patches, IUDs, rings – any of the products.

On the very day my article posted, a 20-year-old woman in Durham, North Carolina lost her life to hormonal birth control. Her father reached out to me and shared the horrible circumstances of his daughter, Alex's death. Up until this point, I thought I had some sense of how tragic it must be to lose your daughter this way, but speaking with Anthony while the grief was still so raw gave me a new understanding of just how deep the pain can run.

Their family was close and usually discussed everything, but Alex had gone to Planned Parenthood on her own. She decided to start birth control in January. Soon thereafter, she began experiencing lower back pains. Her mother took her to an urgent care clinic, where the doctors thought she may have strained her back while working at Whole Foods.

They prescribed muscle relaxers, which seemed to reduce the pain for a while. Then, in early August, the backaches returned with such force that Alex ended up in the Emergency Room. The doctors took X-rays of her upper body and diagnosed her with a lung infection. The antibiotics seemed to help, but Alex still struggled with occasional back pain and her energy levels fluctuated noticeably.

A little over a month had passed since the ER visit. It was a beautiful September morning, and Anthony had stopped by the store to pick up some items on his way to work when he got a call from his wife, Lisa. Alex had collapsed on the driveway. The EMS were there, and he should meet them at Duke University Medical Center right away!

As they waited for news from the team of doctors working to save their daughter's life, Lisa told Anthony about holding Alex on the driveway while they waited for the ambulance. Anthony pictured his daughter laying helplessly in her mother's arms with her fists tightly clenched as she fought for her life. Then, he began to relive all the fond memories of Alex growing up on that same driveway – playing with her dolls, racing her sister, learning to ride her bike.

For the better part of two days, doctors would fight to save Alex. Despite all their efforts, there was little to no brain activity. The neurologist told them the damage to Alex's brain was among the worst he had ever seen. She was pronounced dead on September 27th – eight months after starting birth control.

Alex was active and ate a healthy diet. Her only previous illness was when she got strep throat at four years old. Yet, this active young woman died from pulmonary emboli, blood clots in her lungs.

Anthony said, "They informed us that none of Alex's organs, tissue, or even her eyes were suitable for donation. It was as if a weapon of mass destruction had gone off inside of our daughter's body."

Still stunned and reeling from her death, he sat down at the computer and Googled "blood clots young woman death." Among the results, he found numerous stories of vibrant young women like Alex who had died from taking birth control. His first indication that Alex was taking birth control was after it was already too late to talk to her about it.

Lisa went through Alex's belongings and found her prescription for Levora. At first, Anthony said he felt guilty – like he had let Alex down because he hadn't warned her about the dangers of birth control. Then, he realized that he didn't even know how dangerous they were until it was too late. He said, "It's easy to find articles about how The Pill helps your acne or menstrual pain, but to learn how dangerous these things are you really have to dig and know what you're looking for."

Anthony and Lisa agreed the best way they can honor Alex's memory is to share their story, and hope they can save other families from going through the same tragedy. It's a senseless loss – one that truly should never happen to anyone. Anthony describes how their lives have changed, "Our home was once filled with endless laughter, cooking meals together, practical jokes, and endless hours playing Crazy 8s. Now, our days are filled with therapy appointments, counseling sessions, support group meetings, and learning about bereavement."

Weighing the Risks

When you hear just one story like Alex's, it should be clear that the benefits of hormonal birth control could never outweigh the risks. We're talking about a drug that prevents pregnancy (most of the time) – not one that cures cancer. Let's forget about all the other side effects, and just consider the facts surrounding this one.

There is no debate that all hormonal birth control increases the risk of deadly blood clots. Drug manufacturers have paid billions of dollars to settle lawsuits related to injury and death from these clots (which means they don't have to admit fault, and the families aren't permitted to talk about it). We know for a fact that tens of thousands of women have died from clots related to their birth control since it was first approved by the FDA. My question is how many deaths would it take to be considered unacceptable? How many women would have to die for 'industry experts' to proclaim the benefits no longer outweigh the risks?

CHAPTER 12

Diabetes & Matters of the Heart

Dr. Ernst Rietzschel described his findings as 'startling.' His fellow cardiologists buzzed in agreement after he presented his findings at the American Heart Association 2007 annual meeting. His Ghent University lab in Belgium discovered that women taking hormonal birth control and those who had ever taken them for more than a year have an increased risk of atherosclerosis, plaque build-up, which is most commonly known as hardening of the arteries. And, the risk goes up with the duration of use – up to a 42 percent increased risk with each decade. This was different from the clotting issues most doctors associated with The Pill. They viewed clotting as a short-term side effect that receded after a woman stopped taking synthetic hormones. However, plaque build-up continues long after a woman stops taking birth control and could ultimately lead to deadly consequences like a stroke or heart attack.

Building Blocks

Ideally, medical research is like a set of building blocks. Each new study builds on the foundation of past experiments. While taking us to a new level of understanding, the new study also provides the foundation for the next layer of discovery that lies ahead. Dr. Rietzschel's study contained its own internal set of building blocks. The team initially discovered that women taking hormonal contraceptives had a threefold increase in C-Reactive Protein (CRP) levels. The liver typically increases CRP production in correlation to inflammation levels in the body. Consequently, high CRP levels can act as a marker to indicate the presence of other diseases or conditions associated with inflammation.

Dr. Rietzschel explained how this dramatic rise in CRP levels led to discovering the increased risk of atherosclerosis:

> "This is the first time that this has been documented. It was an accidental finding. We were stunned by the large elevations in CRP that you see in women taking the pill, so we then performed a safety analysis to see whether there was a link between past pill use and atherosclerosis measured by echo in both the carotid and femoral arteries."

Single Layer Research

Dr. Rietzchel's results were groundbreaking, but in many ways, his study exemplifies everything that is wrong in medical research related to hormonal birth control. The ideal building-block metaphor has never really materialized. Rather than resembling a pyramid, the blocks making up birth control research look more like someone let their rambunctious four-year-old brother into the room. These blocks, scattered in disarray, rarely stack to even a second level.

The investigator accurately described his findings as startling, but even more disturbing is that they were discovered entirely by accident. If CRP levels in the subjects hadn't been so ridiculously elevated, the researchers might never have considered the link between The Pill and atherosclerosis – despite the fact that what should have been the foundation for this discovery was laid decades earlier.

A simple Google search reveals that some of the leading factors contributing to atherosclerosis include: high blood pressure, high blood sugar levels, diabetes, and high cholesterol levels. The birth control pill's contribution to each of these conditions was discussed in depth at the Nelson Pill Hearings.

Birth Control and High Blood Pressure

Similar to Dr. Rietzschel, Dr. John Laragh, who testified at the hearings, said that his discovery of the relationship between oral contraceptives and high blood pressure came by chance, "We observed a woman who we knew had normal blood pressure develop rather severe and impressive hypertension several months after starting an oral contraceptive medication."

He confirmed this behavior in several other patients and found that, in most cases, the blood pressure returned to normal after stopping The Pill. After they normalized, two patients who had no previous history of high blood pressure requested to continue with birth control pills. In both cases, their hypertension reappeared when they started taking The Pill again and then disappeared upon terminating the medication.

Dr. Laragh stressed that his trial size was too small to have statistical significance, but this 'rechallenge experiment' convinced him of a cause and effect relationship. Having also observed that some women 'swell up and accumulate salt and water,' he deduced a probable mechanism that could be triggering high blood pressure in birth control patients.

To test his theory, he began measuring certain components of the kidney hormonal system and found that women on birth control experienced enormous increases in renin substrate levels. Renin substrate circulates through the blood and has the capacity to release the hormone, angiotensin. Dr. Laragh described angiotensin as 'the hormone which is the most powerful of all hormones in its capacity to raise the blood pressure.' His suspicions seemed to be confirmed by a 2011 study (40 years later), which found that birth control so significantly elevated angiotensin levels that it could cause false-positive results for a condition which disturbs the balance of sodium and potassium in the blood, known as aldosteronism.

Another block on the floor…

While addressing the big picture at the hearings, Dr. Laragh offered a couple of important caveats for the medical industry. First, he strongly recommended that any patient on birth control be seen by the doctor **every 2 to 3 months** to monitor her blood pressure.

When questioned about such frequent follow-ups, he warned, "We have a responsibility when we have powerful drugs like this; our responsibility is to learn about them, and the second responsibility is to apply the information. Otherwise, we do not have any right to have them on the market."

Blood Sugar Levels and Diabetes

Further evidence that oral contraceptives can cause high blood pressure came in Dr. Philip Corfman's testimony, when he matter-of-factly stated, "It is known that steroids alter the diameter of veins and other blood vessels. These effects are also related to the changes in blood pressure observed in some users of oral contraceptives. Several reports of hypertension have appeared, and there is an increasing body of evidence that there may be a positive relationship."

Dr. Corfman previously headed a task force at the National Institutes of Health. His team combed through nearly 4,000 journal articles and sorted the concerns into more than 20 categories that they felt needed further attention. Much of his testimony focused on birth control's metabolic effects on the body, particularly how the synthetic hormones modified carbohydrate metabolism.

"Recent investigations show that a significant proportion of normal women on these agents appear to handle sugar in an abnormal way." He continued, "Another biologic change of increasing concern is the effect on the way the body handles fat. This effect is closely related to changes in sugar metabolism since fat synthesis is related to insulin levels. The changes which have been observed in fat metabolism simulate levels seen in older individuals and raise concern over the possibility that these alterations may be related to heart disease."

And this was no rare event, Dr. Victor Wynn testified that nearly 1-in-5 young women taking The Pill developed an abnormal glucose tolerance that he named "chemical diabetes."

The Pill and High Cholesterol

Recognizing that there were also abnormalities in the fats circulating in the blood of birth control patients, Dr. Wynn decided to measure triglycerides against a control group. He discovered that "at least one-third of the users had triglyceride values higher than the highest value we found in our control subjects." (NPH 6305) Let that sink in – the woman with the very highest triglyceride values from the control group had numbers lower than one-third of the women on The Pill.

In his beautiful British accent, Dr. Wynn slyly added, "I am sure that there is no need for me to tell an American audience the significance of having your cholesterol levels elevated, since there is so much propaganda in the press, medical, and lay, indicating the importance of having your cholesterol lower, if you can possibly achieve it."

To demonstrate the domino effect of these complications, Dr. Wynn submitted a summary of over 70 references taken from medical literature over the previous 3 years.

"It is by no means exhaustive. But the references are to the association between abnormal glucose metabolism, abnormal insulin levels, and abnormal blood lipid or blood fat levels, and the accelerated development of atherosclerosis."

More blocks on the floor...

Don't Discount Clotting

Respected neurosurgeon, Dr. David Clark testified that the strokes which young women on birth control encountered were different than those seen in older patients. The Pill seemed to trigger a different mechanism, as 'alterations in the normal clotting behavior are certainly present.'

"There is some reason also to believe that there may be changes in the vascular wall itself. It is known that estrogens have an effect on the caliber of veins. In some of the stroke victims who have been studied, there is a peculiar beaded appearance to the walls of the arteries -- not occlusion, but irregularity of outline that suggests there may be edema or other changes in the outer wall of the artery."

Dr. Wynn added, "When you see the abnormalities, these are associated in some curious way with increased incidence of clotting, so that putting the two together, I think it is a reasonable case, but it cannot be proved, and this underlines the great difficulty we have with the contraceptives, that what harm they may do may never in fact be proved."

At the rate we're going, it will certainly never be proved.

Second Level Stuff

However, there is a seed of hope on at least one front. After his study that uncovered the startling link to atherosclerosis, Dr. Rietzschel told Medscape, "It's staggering that for a drug that is being used by 80% of women, there is so little information about the long-term safety. That's really incredible."

Sensing his genuine dismay that so little has been done to understand the safety of hormonal contraceptives, I contacted Dr. Rietzschel to see if he was aware of any subsequent studies building on his atherosclerosis findings. It turns out, his team is in the final stages of a longitudinal study, and he expects the analyses to be published soon.

This is a promising development. Let's just hope no one lets their four-year-old brother into the room.

CHAPTER 13

Birth Control & Breast Cancer:
A Classic Cover Up

"Estrogen is to cancer as fertilizer is to the wheat crop."

It was the first headline-grabbing quote from the Nelson Pill Hearings, and it threw birth control proponents into a tizzy. They complained vociferously that the hearings were alarming women everywhere, and causing them to stop taking The Pill. Sen. Nelson's reply was simple, if women had been warned about the side effects *before* being prescribed, they wouldn't be alarmed hearing about them now.

That one little quote about synthetic estrogens catalyzing cancer and the uproarious reaction exemplify the beauty of the hearings. It really is one of the few times in recent history that the pharmaceutical industry had almost no control over the message.

Fertilizer for Breast Cancer

Before the hearings, Big Pharma managed to suppress knowledge of their product's link to certain cancers, particularly breast cancer. However, in the hearings, those connections came to light and stunned viewers as they tuned into the nightly news.

Here are some of the facts presented by leading physicians at the hearings:

- The American Cancer Society recognized the possible risk of breast cancer as a side effect of hormonal contraceptives as early as 1961. Dr. Max Cutler, Page 6664
- It's imprudent to prescribe oral contraceptives to a woman with a family history of breast cancer. – Dr. Max Cutler, Page 6666
- There was statistical evidence that breast cancer associated with pill takers in the FDA files had been dramatically underreported. – James Duffy, Page 6069
- All human carcinogens are latent. And, it could take 10 to 20 years of patient history to determine the cancer impact. Dr. Victor Wynn, Page 6309
- Not only had the synthetic hormones used in The Pill been proven to cause breast cancer in all five species of animals that had been injected with it, but it also caused the very rare condition of breast cancer in human males. Dr. Hugh Davis, Page 5927
- There should be no chronic use of The Pill. It is a cancer time bomb with a fuse that could be 15 to 20 years. Dr. Max Cutler, Page 6669

Perhaps the most crucial statement as it relates to us today was this from Dr. Hugh Davis:

"Now, there are some 75 to 80,000 women in this country per year who are developing diagnosed carcinoma of the breast. If the chronic taking of steroid hormones eventually increased this by only 10 percent, we would have a very, very hazardous situation on our hands..." (NPH, Page 5931)

I know how easily our eyes can glaze over when someone starts quoting statistics, but please pay attention to these numbers! In 1970, 1 out of every 20 women developed breast cancer sometime during her life according to Dr. Max Cutler. (NPH, Page 6666) You just read that Dr. Davis said it would be 'a very, very hazardous situation' if we saw a 10 percent increase over the 75 to 80,000 diagnoses each year.

Today, we have witnessed a **210 percent increase!** 1 in every 8 women will develop breast cancer in her life. Over 246,000 cases of breast cancer will be diagnosed this year. If the vastly underestimated 10 percent was considered very hazardous, then our reality hit a level of hazard that defies description.

Message Control

The hearings also pulled back the curtain on how the pharmaceutical industry manipulated the message to the media and the medical community.

In 1967, *Child & Family Quarterly* started a section called, "Recent Setbacks in Medicine," which seemed to be largely inspired by the introduction of hormonal birth control. They wrote, "The Pill quickly became big business, so that drug manufacturers began to manipulate professional opinion at an early date, stressing the wonders of the Pill and minimizing its dangers."

Speaking to this point, Sen. Nelson pointed out the conflicting statements of Dr. Louis Hellman, who chaired the FDA's study on The Pill. He said:

> "I doubt whether there is one person, one doctor in a thousand in this country who is aware that [Dr. Hellman] said, 'Now, in discussing the chairman's report, the right statement has to be made. We cannot just hide behind rhetoric. We are going to have to say something, and we have an opinion; that these are not safe, and the Commissioner might have to take them off the market if he believes this. We can say these are safe and our scientific data did not really permit that kind of statement.'"

Their official statement ended up being that hormonal contraceptives were "Safe within the intent of the legislation." This strangely mitigated reference to Kefauver-Harris legislation was all the pharmaceutical industry needed because it contained the word 'safe.' Despite admitting that the committee believed The Pill wasn't safe, Dr. Hellman then hit the media circuit to reassure women that it was.

Cures Not Causes

At Big Pharma, manipulation is the modus operandi, but no example is more disgusting and deplorable as Breast Cancer Awareness Month (BCAM). I know that sounds shocking, but consider this. If an organization started promoting Lung Cancer Awareness Month, but they never mentioned smoking, would you think there was something fishy in the air?

For all this 'search for the cure,' there is little to no talk of preventive measures. There's a good reason for that. Jim Hightower explains it perfectly in his book, *There's Nothing in the Middle of the Road but Yellow Stripes and Dead Armadillos*:

> "Breast Cancer Awareness Month is a front that was conceived, funded, and launched in 1985 by a British conglomerate with a name that could come straight out of a Batman comic book: Imperial Chemical Industries (ICI). But the $14-billion-a-year multinational behemoth is all too real. It is among the world's largest makers of pesticides, plastics, pharmaceuticals, and paper. "Organochlorines R Us" could legitimately be its slogan."

In 1993, Monte Paulsen of the *Detroit Metro Times* wrote, "ICI has been the sole financial sponsor of BCAM since the event's inception. Altogether, the company has spent 'several million dollars' on the project, according to a spokeswoman. In return, ICI has been allowed to approve – or veto – every poster, pamphlet, and advertisement BCAM uses."

ICI's pharmaceutical division, Zeneca Group PLC later split off to become AstraZeneca, taking Breast Cancer Awareness Month with them. Kudos to Mr. Paulsen for digging into this. AstraZeneca's 'ownership' of BCAM is typically framed as being purely philanthropic. They can't lose. They actually strategized a way to make breast cancer a win-win situation for their shareholders.

Jim Hightower continues:

"It gets gooier. Zeneca's pharmaceutical arm is also the maker of Nolvadex, the leading drug used in breast cancer treatment. Nolvadex is a highly controversial drug – it does not cure existing breast cancer, but it can help stop it from spreading in some women who are diagnosed early; however, it can also cause blood clots, uterine cancer, and liver cancer in those who take it... What a racket this company has going! It makes billions selling industrial organochlorines linked to breast cancer, it finances its BCAM front to divert public attention from cancer causes to cancer detection, then it sells Nolvadex to those who are detected."

Industrial waste and toxic chemicals may be responsible for the spike in breast cancer, and synthetic estrogens may be the fertilizer that feeds it, but, ultimately, it's Big Pharma that's spreading the manure.

Same Old Same Old

Despite the incredibly high incidence of breast cancer, most people (including medical professionals) have bought into the storyline that the link between birth control and breast cancer is old news – a problem that was resolved by the new generation of birth control pills and devices.

This, of course, is another fallacy perpetuated by the drug industry's PR machine. Whenever bad news gets close to sticking to birth control, they simply reformulate the product and deem it safe (without any real science to back up the claim). And, we take their word for it – only to be made to look like fools...again.

In December 2017, the *New York Times* reported on a massive study that followed 1.8 million Danish women for 10 years. It found that women on hormonal contraceptives were 20 percent more likely to develop breast cancer. This was the first significant study to include modern devices like hormonal IUD's as well as progestin-only devices.

As unsettling as the findings were, the verbiage used in the *Times* article proves the most disturbing. The article quotes Dr. Marisa Weiss, an oncologist who founded breastcancer.org. She says, "This is an important study because we had no idea how the modern day pills compared... and we didn't know anything about IUD's. Gynecologists just <u>assumed</u> that a lower dose of hormone meant a lower risk of cancer. But the same elevated risk is there."

To understand just how broadly accepted the assumptions about birth control were (and still are, despite the release of this study), consider these phrases, all taken from that same article:

"...upends widely held assumptions about modern contraceptives."

"Many women have believed that newer hormonal contraceptives are much safer than those taken by their mothers or grandmothers..."

"...this study is the first to examine the risks associated with current formulations."

"There was a hope that the contemporary preparations would be associated with lower risk." (from a professor of medicine at the University of Oxford)

"What really surprised the researchers was that the increased risk was not confined to women using oral contraceptive pills, but also was seen in women using implanted intrauterine devices, or IUD's, that contain the hormone progestin."

Even the study's lead author, Lina S. Morch from the University of Copenhagen, thought the new formulations were going to be proven safer, "We did actually expect we would find a smaller increase in risk because today we have lower doses of estrogen in hormone contraceptives, so it was surprising that we found this association... It is a very clear picture for us, very convincing."

Convincing, yes, but it really shouldn't have been surprising. Only three years earlier, the National Cancer Institute funded a study at the Fred Hutchinson Cancer Research Center in Seattle, which found that women who had taken certain modern birth control pills within the past year faced a 50 percent increased risk of breast cancer.

Prior to that, the *Mayo Clinic Proceedings* published a meta-analysis of 34 major studies. The researchers discovered that in 90 percent of the studies, women who took The Pill before having children faced a 44 percent increased risk of getting breast cancer before the age of 50. However, the lead investigator, Dr. Chris Kahlenborn may have made his most astute observation during an interview with the *National Catholic Register*:

"[Dr. Kahlenborn] suggests many researchers, particularly in the U.S., are 'petrified' of telling the truth about the link between breast cancer and the pill for fear of losing their funding.

"What's more, media outlets typically try to ignore any harm caused by the pill because they don't want to offend their pharmaceutical-company advertisers. For example, the media virtually ignored the Mayo findings.

"'It's disgusting,' Kahlenborn declared. 'Women are dying. We put our study out there. Almost nobody knew about it, because it was basically buried by the media.'"

CHAPTER 14

Permanent Sterilization

I vividly recall the most unexpected reaction I got when I told a friend that we were pregnant with our daughter. He asked me not to mention it in front of his wife yet. He explained that she was in the midst of an emotional crisis. Their attempts to conceive had been unsuccessful, and the doctors suspected she had fertility issues.

As he shared more about their ordeal, he said that they wondered if her years on birth control could have had anything to do with it. I agreed that it seemed like a logical possibility. (This was over a decade ago, long before I cared one way or the other about The Pill). We discussed how odd it would be if birth control could cause fertility issues, that we had never heard anything about it. And, like so many 'common sense' questions about hormonal birth control, we shrugged it off.

Fertility Fatigue

That conversation faded into the recesses of my mind until I found myself at a medical conference a few years later. The conference focused on several inflammatory diseases. I noticed a trend in how carefully the presenters handled the subject of prescribing prednisone, a synthetic corticosteroid. Anytime it was recommended as a treatment, the presenter always included the typical disclaimers - 'go with the lowest dose possible,' 'minimize the duration,' and 'taper the patient off the drug'... I was familiar with adrenal fatigue and understood their motivation.

Even low doses of prednisone can upset the delicate endocrine system. Our body responds to the influx of those synthetic steroids by reducing the production of cortisol and other adrenal hormones. Extended use of the drug or suddenly stopping the medication can cause an adrenal crisis, and, in some cases, the damage is permanent.

As I contemplated how this flood of synthetic hormones overrides the production of natural hormones, I recalled the previous conversation with my friend. Over the next few days, I struck up conversations with some of the doctors attending the meeting. I told them I was curious about the frequent mention of prednisone and how the presenters were clearly concerned about preventing adrenal fatigue. Then, I drew a parallel and asked a simple question, "Should we have the same concern about how the synthetic hormones in birth control may be affecting the production of *those* hormones?"

Each doctor had virtually the same response. First, a perplexed look crossed their face. Then, they admitted, "That's a good question. I never really thought about it."

Delayed Fertility

That's a fitting response because doctors generally don't think about it. As side effects go, delayed fertility and even infertility rank low on the totem pole of consequences tied to hormonal birth control. Certainly, doctors are not going to give it the attention they might give other ailments caused by birth control, like breast cancer or strokes. However, the problem isn't that infertility has been neglected or underestimated so much as it's been completely dismissed.

Our cultural paradigm tells women that planning their family is as easy as 1-2-3.

Step 1: Take The Pill until you're ready for kids.

Step 2: Stop taking The Pill.

Step 3: Start your family.

But, it isn't always that easy. Since doctors are unaware of the connection, they frequently assure patients that their birth control couldn't have caused infertility. A persistent patient might turn to Google, but those results are just as confusing. One top hit says, "There's no evidence that long-term use of the birth control pill interferes with fertility," while another states, "It can take a few extra months to start menstrual cycles..." but confidently adds that "birth control doesn't hurt your chances of having a baby in the future."

As Old as The Pill

When I began researching birth control in earnest, my focus was on autoimmune disease, but it didn't take long to discover that infertility was actually one of the original concerns about The Pill. In fact, Barbara Seaman devoted an entire chapter to it in her famous book, *The Doctors' Case Against The Pill*.

She wrote, "It is no longer just a vague worry but an established fact that a certain number of women simply do not start having their periods again after they stop taking the pill. Others have irregular or scanty periods. In either case, they may find that they cannot conceive. They are sterile."

She introduced readers to Dr. M. James Whitelaw, a fertility expert who fought through bitter attacks from some in the medical community to publish a report on a phenomenon he called "oversuppression syndrome" in The *Journal of the American Medical Association* (JAMA) in February 1966. After its publication, one well-known doctor responded, "Now, Dr. Whitelaw is regarded as a prophet. We all admire his courage and persistence in smoking this thing out."

When the Nelson Pill Hearings rolled around in 1970, they called on Dr. Whitelaw to testify. He explained "oversuppression syndrome" in layman terms, "Any part of the body which is not used, or little used, over a protracted period leads to so-called 'disuse atrophy.'" In this case, the atrophy occurs in the lining of the uterus, and Dr. Whitelaw estimated that it contributed to a 10 percent increase in the rate of infertility.

Dr. Roy Hertz, an FDA advisor, subsequently testified that the introduction of hormonal birth control also disturbed the balance of microscopic activity in the endometrium. These structural and functional abnormalities sometimes lead to cancer of the endometrium, but they also contribute to an atrophy of the endometrium that sometimes leads to permanent infertility.

Recent history hasn't given us many studies that examine the link between hormonal contraceptives and infertility. However, a 1997 study came to the somewhat dubious conclusion that, "The return of fertility for women who discontinue oral contraceptives takes longer as compared with women who discontinue other methods of contraception."

Modern research may have dropped the ball on "oversuppression syndrome," but it has uncovered some other serious fertility-related concerns. In Chapter 22, we will look at how the fertility crisis extends beyond just the women taking The Pill to include men and even other species.

Oh, and the next time a friend wonders out loud whether birth control could have contributed to their infertility, the short answer is YES.

CHAPTER 15

Depression & Mood Disorders:
Trivialized Side Effects

Doctors frequently dismiss irritability and depression as minor side effects of birth control – a mere inconvenience that can easily be treated. All you need is another prescription. In fact, some doctors will prescribe an anti-depressant for virtually *any* side effect triggered by The Pill.

Trivializing changes in the brain's chemistry, or for that matter, any of the body's chemistry is a dangerous game of roulette. It's akin to the early days of The Pill when doctors recognized that synthetic hormones altered the chemistry in a woman's breasts. Rather than be concerned about what these changes might mean in the long run, they turned it into a marketing point. It makes your breasts fuller! Only after it was undeniably linked to breast cancer did they acknowledge the changes *could be* cause for concern.

In fact, psychological concerns were also raised early on. Earlier in this book, you read that Barbara Seaman sent a copy of her landmark book, *The Doctors' Case Against the Pill* to Sen. Gaylord Nelson in hopes of inspiring what would later become known as the Nelson Pill Hearings. Her six-page letter accompanying the book detailed many of the concerns expressed by physicians. In the letter as in her book, Ms. Seaman masterfully mixed the anecdotal with the science to make her case. She wrote:

> "The pill's effect on personality is a problem that deeply concerns my husband, a psychiatrist. It has long been known that these powerful hormones make some women irritable and some depressed. It has long been maintained by some doctors (and not only psychiatrists) that suicide, not blood clots, may, in fact, be the leading cause of pill death."

First Generation Depression

A smattering of uncomfortable laughter danced through the Senate chambers when Mayo-trained, Philip Ball M.D. testified on the side effects of birth control at the hearings:

> "In a fair number of these women, the husband will call me separately, and say, 'My God, do something about my wife, she has just turned into a bitch.' Or the mother or mother-in-law [will call], but these problems are often stated by other members of the

family who have observed a total change of personality." (NPH Page 6499)

Family members weren't the only ones noticing these changes. A large-scale Swedish study revealed that 'psychiatric reasons' was the primary reason given by women for stopping birth control. (NPH Page 6452)
At one end of the spectrum, symptoms were compared to 'constant pre-menstrual tension.' But, the other end of the spectrum skewed much darker. It included suicidal and even murderous tendencies.

Dr. Francis Kane was a gynecologist from the University of North Carolina who was among the first to document psychological changes in patients. He also testified at the hearings. He shared the results of a British study, which paralleled his findings that one out of every three pill users studied showed depressive personality changes, and a little more than one out of every 20 became suicidal. He added that women on birth control had 'distinctly higher scores,' meaning not only were more of them getting depressed, but the depression they were experiencing was greater than non-pill users. (NPH Page 6456)

The Serious Side of Side Effects

In her book, Barbara Seaman described the behavioral changes women experience on The Pill:

"A few pill users have become so hostile, suspicious and delusional that they have seriously thought of murdering – or have actually attempted to murder – their own husbands and children. Others attempt to commit suicide and some have succeeded."

Dr. Harold Williams also authored a book, *Pregnant or Dead*, which came out the same year. In it, he attempted to quantify some of the collateral damage associated with The Pill. One of his most shocking finds came when he compiled suicide statistics from the most recent year (1967) and compared them with statistics from 1961 (representing the last year before birth control became commonplace).

The increases were dramatically higher than their male counterparts. Dr. Williams' conservative estimate was that an additional 223 women in the United States had committed suicide in that one year due to The Pill. Here's what the percentages looked like by age:

Percent Change Rate

Age	Change
15-19	+93%
20-24	+100%
25-29	+54%
30-34	+74%
35-39	+37%
40-44	+41%

Even one of The Pill's developers, Dr. Celso-Ramon Garcia, had this to say in the March 1968 issue of *JAMA*:

"Relatively little is known about various effects, especially those on personality and emotions... The fact that many questions remain unanswered points out the necessity for further investigation into the areas of emotional responses to the use of hormonal contraceptives."

Still the Same

As with so many other complications, subsequent generations of birth control didn't eliminate the problem. Using the Danish National Patient Registry, researchers in Denmark conducted a cohort study of one million young women in 2016. They discovered that women taking hormonal birth control were 70 percent more likely to develop depression. The greatest likelihood of depression was found in women using non-oral forms of contraceptive, with women using the transdermal patch expressing a two-fold increased risk.

One year later, in 2017, the same Danish researchers released the results of an even more alarming study that suggested (just as researchers concluded in the late 1960s) that the depression these women experience is more intense than that of women who have never taken hormonal birth control. The study, published in the *American Journal of Psychiatry*, reported that women on birth control more than tripled their risk of committing suicide!

Below the Surface

As dramatic and dangerous as these behavioral changes sometimes are, recent studies suggest they could merely be the most obvious and immediate short-range psychiatric complications. Unfortunately, the less obvious, long-range complications could ultimately be just as damaging.

In the Name of The Pill

A lot is left to learn about the complex role of hormones in the various functions of the human body, but scientists do recognize that estrogens play a key role in the immune system. Natural estrogen, estradiol, activates the immune system to provide an increased level of protection against infectious disease for women, especially during their reproductive years. However, the introduction of birth control or hormone replacement therapy into the system creates a cascade of problems. First, it floods the body with synthetic estrogen, which is molecularly different from natural estrogens. The body reacts to the overabundance of these potent chemicals by cutting back on the production of natural estradiol.

In a healthy woman's body, the first noticeable sign that estradiol has triggered the immune system is typically inflammation. Estradiol combines with receptor cells in the immune system to produce cytokines, which regulate inflammation. However, synthetic estrogens frequently throw this delicate system out of balance and confuse the immune system in ways we will revisit in a moment.

Often times, the production (and overproduction) of cytokines can be localized within the body. Studies have shown that synthetic estrogen contributes to overproduction of at least two cytokines in the central nervous system: interleukin 6 (IL-6, which we will visit again in Chapter 18 on multiple sclerosis), and interferon-gamma. A recent study published in *JAMA Psychiatry* concluded that brain inflammation was 30 percent higher in clinically depressed patients, while another study linked increased interferon-gamma secretion to major depression.

Not Immune to Depression

Groundbreaking new research from the University of Virginia has begun to reveal how the immune system influences mental disorders and neurological diseases. The headline on *Science Alert* in July 2016 read, "Freaky New Evidence Suggests Your Immune System Could Be Controlling Your Behaviour." In the article, lead researcher, Jonathan Kipnis, speculates, "Part of our personality may actually be dictated by the immune system."

The article goes on to explain:

"The molecule in question is called interferon gamma, and it's usually released by the immune system when it comes into contact with a pathogen, such as a virus or bacteria.

"This type of immune response is part of the adaptive immune system, which learns to keep an eye out for nasty germs - and up until last year, it was thought to be isolated from the brain as a result of the blood-brain barrier. "

The discovery of meningeal lymphatic vessels that connect the brain to the immune system also came from the Kipnis lab. This revolutionary discovery changed nearly everything neuroscientists believed about the blood-brain barrier and created a whole new perspective on the interaction of the brain with the immune system. This missing link suggests the neurological consequences of birth control could run much deeper than interferon-gamma and depression.

Establishing this physical connection to the brain makes it easier to connect the dots on other previously demonstrated relationships with mental disorders and brain diseases. It suddenly seems less mysterious that women who take hormonal birth control are 50 percent more likely to develop a glioma brain tumor.

It also makes sense that inflammation is present, and the brain's immune cells are hyperactive in schizophrenia patients. Is it any wonder that patients with autoimmune disease have a 45 percent increased risk of schizophrenia, or that they are 20 percent more likely to develop dementia later in life?

Autoimmunity Attacks the Brain

Our focus doesn't officially shift to autoimmunity until the next chapter, but let's take a moment to look a little closer at that relationship between autoimmunity and schizophrenia.

Autoimmune encephalitis (also known as anti-NMDA receptor encephalitis) typically affects the brain in a younger population, and (like most AI diseases) it targets women much more than men. Studies in animal models have shown an increased production of IL-6 associated with this disease, as well.

Autoimmune encephalitis is a relatively rare disease – or at least it is a rarely diagnosed disease. The disease was first identified by Dr. Joseph Dalmau in the early 2000s. At a recent symposium in Houston, doctors offered a lowball estimate that at least 3.2 million Americans currently diagnosed with schizophrenia actually suffer from undiagnosed autoimmune encephalitis. Dr. Dalmau said, "These patients develop symptoms that can fool any psychiatrist."

The *Houston Chronicle* reported on the symposium, "During his presentation at Methodist Friday, Dalmau played a video of a woman lying on her back in a hospital, mouth twitching as she stared vacantly at the ceiling. Then he played a video of her not long after beginning immunotherapy treatment, walking down the hall of the hospital. And then another, weeks later, showing her sitting up, smiling and talking normally."

Back to the Future

One of the things that most concerned doctors in the early days of birth control was that they didn't know what they didn't know. They saw things were changing. They witnessed certain side effects and complications, but they feared the things they weren't yet seeing.

They knew The Pill hadn't been sufficiently tested and were concerned about what side effects might be flying below their radar. Here's what one doctor shared with Barbara Seaman:

> "Dr. Ayd told us, that some physicians were still giving patients tranquilizers to counteract pill-caused psychiatric symptoms. Some drugs, taken in combination, produce untoward effects in some people. Researchers were learning that the combination of the pill and certain psychiatric drugs could produce a broad range of dangerous and unpleasant effects. Among these were tremor and rigidity as in Parkinson's disease."... "It needs to be emphasized that if you give a patient one drug and

counteract it with another, there is a rising curve of adverse reactions."

Dr. Ayd was obviously concerned about the practice of giving psychiatric drugs to treat Pill-induced symptoms. Unfortunately, fifty years later, that practice has become the standard.

CHAPTER 16

An Introduction to Autoimmune Disease

The industrialized world finds itself in the midst of a full-blown epidemic. In the United States alone, over 23 million people suffer from an autoimmune disease (AI). Collectively, their incidence is higher than that of cancer or heart disease.

As a classification, AI consists of nearly 100 disparate diseases. At first glance, many of these ailments may seem to have nothing in common. Yet, the common factor that unifies them under the AI umbrella is that they are each the product of a renegade immune system attacking the body's healthy tissue. These attacks manifest as a host of diseases affecting virtually every part of the body.

My Introduction to AI

My introduction to AI came from a man known as the Father of Autoimmune Disease, Dr. Noel Rose. He first hypothesized the idea of the body's immune system attacking itself in the late 50s. He developed the theory and came up with the name autoimmune disease while studying Hashimoto's Thyroiditis in rabbits.

It was a lecture by Dr. Rose that sparked my interest in birth control research. That evening, the amiable, elder statesman explained the basics of autoimmunity. He said we knew from the beginning that estrogens probably played a vital role in autoimmunity because of the role they play in a woman's immune system, plus the fact that nearly 80 percent of all diagnoses were (and are) women.

He explained that patients must be genetically predisposed to contract an autoimmune disease, but stressed that environmental triggers are the real key to activating the condition in a patient.

He described T cells as soldiers of the immune system. When our body's natural estrogens attach to T cell receptors, the soldiers are armed and have their marching orders. The estrogen essentially points out the invader and triggers the command to attack. But when disruptive agents that mimic natural estrogen enter our body (known as endocrine disruptors), they attach to the receptors. Suddenly, the soldier is armed but doesn't know what to attack. This can cause the immune system to start a battle with our body's healthy tissue, resulting in the triggering of an AI.

Although Dr. Rose didn't insinuate The Pill was to blame, his lecture inspired me to dig deeper into what I have grown to believe is the most prolific endocrine disruptor on the planet, a chemical that was quite literally designed to mimic natural estrogen in the body - hormonal contraceptives.

No Prototype

There is no prototypical AI disease. Estrogen's role isn't always easily identified, especially in those diseases with more balanced gender ratios. But, for those that strongly discriminate against women, it clearly plays a pivotal role, and that role can change from disease to disease.

For example, some diseases, like lupus, occur more frequently in the reproductive years and seem to be triggered by high levels of estrogen. However, the onset of diseases like rheumatoid arthritis tend to occur later in life and seem to be triggered by the absence of estrogen. Then, you have paradoxical diseases like multiple sclerosis, which seem to be triggered by, but also temporarily relieved by the flood of estrogens from birth control. This relief comes at a hefty price, as we will see.

Genetic Versus Environmental

The first show I worked with my friend, Jack, was a pretty relaxed gig. He noticed that I pulled out my laptop and began writing every time we hit a lull. When he asked what I was working on, he was fascinated to learn I was writing an article on autoimmune disease. His wife struggles with multiple AI diseases. We discussed the horrible toll it had taken on his young wife, how her symptoms had reacted to her recent pregnancy, and how she was coping with subsequent fatigue while raising a young child.

When I shared my theory with him that The Pill had been largely responsible for the sharp rise in AI diseases over the past 50 years, he said, "Not with my wife, she was diagnosed with her first autoimmune disease at the age of 17, long before she started any birth control."

I told him that it wasn't my belief that all autoimmune cases were caused by The Pill, but that I was always interested to hear the timing in relation to when they started birth control and its effect on their ailment.

The next morning he said that he had told his wife about our conversation and that she actually had started on birth control when she was 17, not long before her first symptoms. Of course, anecdotal stories like this don't prove the theory, but I have encountered too many similar stories and dug up too much supportive science to believe they are coincidental.

The funny thing is I worked with Jack again a few weeks later. He told me that his wife had been to her doctor, and "after talking to him, she was convinced her diseases were not caused by birth control. The doctor had told her they were genetic."

This has almost become a mantra for me, and you will see it more than once in this book, but it bears repeating - all AI diseases are genetic in the sense that you must be genetically predisposed in order to contract the disease. However, as I had learned from Dr. Rose, environmental triggers are critical to activating the disease.

Studies focused on identical twins have confirmed the importance of environmental triggers. If any disease

An Introduction to Autoimmune Disease

were purely genetic and attacked one twin, by their very nature, it would strike the other sibling. However, AI studies have found these illnesses only struck both twins 24 percent of the time.

Diverse Commonality

Despite the differences in the broad scope of diseases that fall under the AI umbrella, there is evidence of a robust underlying bond. One in every four autoimmune patients will be diagnosed with another AI disease. But, the connection expands beyond what's been labeled as multiple autoimmune syndrome.

The disparity of the various autoimmune diseases made it difficult for doctors to recognize what was happening. Focused on patients within their own specialty, physicians witnessed growing outbreaks of specific diseases for years but failed to make the connection that they were related. As Donna Jackson Nakazawa, author of The Autoimmune Epidemic put it, "There was no one standing on the mountaintop saying, 'Wow, look what's happening in all these valleys.'"

The fragmentation and compartmentalization of modern western medicine seem to have obscured their ability to connect the dots. Consequently, it sometimes takes years for a patient to be correctly diagnosed.

Honestly, very little is still known about AIs in the grand scheme of things. This we do know. Hormones are powerful chemical messengers that play a role in just about every process our bodies perform. Even though we don't know precisely how these messengers work or exactly what their role is in the immune system, we should know enough by now to leave them alone and to try not to throw them out of balance.

The following chapters focus on specific AIs, but it is best not to think of them as mutually exclusive. Our bodies are not vacuums; they are machines. Problems that arise tend to affect the broader system, not just engage in an isolated attack.

In fact, the preceding chapters on the original threats make the point for why we shouldn't even consider AI in exclusive terms. For example, in Chapter 12 we saw that the increase of C-Reactive Protein and elevated blood sugar levels that contribute to diabetes also play a role in plaque build-up and heart disease. In Chapter 15, we saw how The Pill causes the body to overproduce interleukin-6 (IL-6), which likely contributes to depression. In Chapter 18, we will see how that same overproduction of IL-6 may trigger multiple sclerosis in those who are genetically predisposed.

Once you break free from the compartmentalization of modern medicine, it becomes much easier to say, "Wow, look what's happening in all these valleys!"

CHAPTER 17

Systemic Lupus Erythematosus

Half a century ago, the National Institutes of Health sponsored a study on the metabolic effects of hormonal contraceptives. In the committee's final report, Dr. Hilton Salhanick wrote:

"These accumulated data and others suggest that no tissue or organ system is free from a biological, functional, and/or morphological effect of contraceptive steroids." [NPH, Page 6567]

Fifty years later, the words of Dr. Noel Rose, the Father of Autoimmune Disease, rang with an eerie familiarity as he (almost proudly) proclaimed, "There is an autoimmune disease for every organ in the body."

Atypical Autoimmunity

There's no such thing as a typical autoimmune disease. Even in their commonalities, they like to express their individuality. Like cousins determined to be different, each AI has a unique relationship with estrogen. Researchers examining the differences in multiple sclerosis (MS) and systemic lupus erythematosus (SLE) found that rising estradiol levels create a protective effect in an MS patient, while it provokes and enhances flares in a lupus patient. They explained the complex distinctions:

> "The effects of sex hormones (such as estrogens) on autoimmune diseases cannot be generalized and is context/disease-dependent. It is not surprising that the outcome of estrogen-mediated autoimmune responses is different among autoimmune diseases since estrogens affect all cells of the immune system, and the triggering and pathogenic mechanisms are varied among different diseases."

Teams of scientists are just beginning to identify the complex stew of variables that contribute to AI diseases. Identification of the specific T-regs (a type of T cell that modulates the immune system), receptor molecules on T cells, and cytokines (proteins that play an important role in cell signaling) will help unlock the greatest mysteries of each AI disease. For now, researchers all seem to agree on one thing - estrogen affects EVERY cell in the immune system. One unfortunate stumbling block in this process is the generic use of the term 'estrogen.' The word is frequently used interchangeably to describe estradiol (estrogen produced naturally within the body) and the synthetic estrogens used in birth control or hormone replacement therapy. These synthetic molecules are very different from natural estradiol, and consequently, have very different effects on our immune systems. We can see the potential impact of synthetic estrogens by examining the evolution of lupus.

The Mysterious Evolution of Lupus

Imagine you're a rheumatologist. You developed your foundational understanding of lupus in medical school, but you really define lupus by what you've seen first-hand in your practice. Everything you know about the onset of disease, the typical patient, when it flares, and when it doesn't is based on (and somewhat limited by) your time in practice.

Now, forget everything you know about lupus, and look at it through the eyes of a physician practicing in the late 1960s.

Everything Dr. Giles Bole Jr. knew about lupus from his time in practice was being challenged. Events he had first classified as anomalies grew more frequent. Through conversations with concerned colleagues, he realized he wasn't the only one feeling uneasy about birth control pills. Even some medical journals started doubting the 'miracle pills' that had been on the market for less than a decade. An editorial in the October 1969 edition of *The Lancet* said, "The wisdom of administering such compounds to healthy women for many years must be seriously questioned." [NPH p. 6109]

Dr. Bole took up research that landed him before Congress at the Nelson Pill Hearings. He described the phenomenon of young women contracting SLE, a rare disorder that was even rarer in young patients. He presented several examples of patients who developed symptoms within the first few months of starting The Pill. In many cases, the symptoms reversed when the women stopped taking the synthetic hormones. Scientists at that time were already aware of certain medications causing drug-induced lupus erythematosus (DILE), but this was different because it was happening in young women, and in many cases, the symptoms were irreversible.

These weren't just isolated cases in Dr. Bole's lab. Later in the hearings, Dr. Herbert Ratner estimated that one of every 2,000 birth control users developed lupus. [NPH p. 6737] (Today, the typical rate is estimated to be 1 in 10,000). Dr. Bole speculated that the synthetic compounds in birth control were to blame, saying that the ability to crossover between synthetic and natural hormones had limitations. He added, "I believe that it is clear to all of us that additional long-term studies relating to the biological effects of these compounds are extremely important."

Lupus Today

A report published in *Arthritis and Rheumatism* in 1999 concluded that the incidence of lupus had tripled in the past forty years. The CDC offers a conservative estimate of 322,000 patients currently suffering from SLE in the US, while the Lupus Foundation of America estimates the number to be 1.5 million. Either way, something sparked this once rare disease. And, 90 percent of those suffering are women.

In 2009, scientists from McGill University in Montreal released the results of a massive population study. They collected data on 1.7 million women and found that women on oral contraceptives were 50 percent more likely to develop lupus. The greatest risk was in the first three months when there was a 2.5-fold increased risk.

Studies like this give us overwhelming preliminary evidence that hormonal contraceptives play a role in causing lupus. Unfortunately, we aren't much closer to confirming the suspicions today than we were when Dr. Bole testified.

The State of Lupus Research

Instead of developing more extensive trials to investigate The Pill's role in triggering lupus, researchers gave us the Safety of Estrogens in Lupus Erythematosus National Assessment (SELENA) trial, which resulted in the study director writing, "Should oral contraceptives be prescribed in SLE? In the last five years, we have come a long way. The answer today is frequently 'yes', whereas before, the answer was almost always 'never.'"

In fact, the trial seemed to be designed for the sole purpose of reversing the answer to a 'yes' – to identify a new market of hormonal contraceptive users, a subset of SLE patients who could 'safely' take The Pill.

The trial's summary claimed, "The results of the study will show whether it is safe for women with SLE to use the pill." This is a very broad statement given the selective group of only 183 SLE patients who participated in the trial. To be included, investigators required a patient to have inactive or stable disease requiring less than 0.5 mg prednisone per kg of body weight per day over a 2-year period. They excluded patients with blood pressure higher than 145/95, any history of thrombosis, APL antibodies, hepatic dysfunction, diabetes, or complicated migraines. We're talking about a very select group of healthy SLE patients being tested. Therefore, it is not surprising their trial concluded 'that oral contraceptives do not increase the risk of flare among women with SLE whose disease is stable.' Of course, for those so inclined, it is easy enough to drop the mitigating phrase from the end of that sentence and proclaim The Pill to be safe for SLE patients, period.

The Art of Deception

Studies like these muddy the waters. They give the impression that birth control won't affect lupus but read any lupus forum and you will find entries like this one:

> "...At this point I decided to stop my birth control because I felt my body needed a break from medications. Within 6 months my hair was growing back, my fatigue went away, as well as the severe swelling. I was able to workout again and live my life! This was 4 years ago and I feel great. I still have flare ups, but it is not constant like it used to be. Recently I tried going on a different type of birth control (lowest hormone levels offered called Loestrin Fe) and had the same side effects within 8 months. I try to find info on birth control and lupus symptoms and how they correlate but have had no luck. Does anyone else have this problem or heard of birth control doing this? My doctor isn't convinced that it is the birth control, but I think it is. Instead of taking me off the birth

control, he is giving me anti-depressants to help me sleep so I'm not tired all the time. "

Let me take a moment to punctuate the absurdity of her situation. She went off The Pill, and her symptoms improved dramatically. Years later, she tried a new formulation of birth control, and the symptoms returned. BUT, her medical professional doesn't think it's The Pill. So, he's prescribing anti-depressants instead! I really wish I could say I've never heard anything like this before, but I have. And, I've heard variations of the scenario so frequently that I'm beginning to think this may be the new standard of practice.

It doesn't help that the website for a major lupus advocacy group contains information like this:

"Many women have more lupus symptoms before menstrual periods and/or during pregnancy when estrogen production is high. This may indicate that estrogen somehow regulates the severity of lupus. However, no causal effect has been proven between estrogen, or any other hormone, and lupus. And, studies of women with lupus taking estrogen in either birth control pills or as postmenopausal therapy have shown no increase in significant disease activity."

No mention of the SLE needing to be stable – no mention of serious secondary symptoms to take into consideration - just straight up, "If you have lupus, The Pill is no cause for concern." Doctors five years prior surely had some reason they were telling lupus patients they should 'never' take The Pill.

It's true 'no causal effect has been proven,' but only because the drug manufacturers don't want it to be proven. Look up virtually any illness that has been linked to birth control, and you will find someone friendly to the drug companies (and the lupus advocacy group certainly receives enough funding from drug companies to fall into this category) who's willing to throw out the 'not proven' argument. In his 1969 book, *Pregnant or Dead*, Dr. Harold Williams described how drug companies were already employing this strategy to deny the link to serious clotting issues. He said they would express the desire for more complete data, while they took steps to thwart the compilation of such data.

What's the Point?

The most important point is this – trust your questions more than the answers. If an answer doesn't ring true, you don't have to accept it just because it came from your doctor or some online expert. Make sure they are hearing your concerns. If necessary, seek a second opinion.

I have spoken with women who were convinced their AI must have been caused by The Pill… until a doctor convinced them otherwise. Afterward, they were convinced it was genetic. Once again - of course, it's genetic! Estimates say that one in every four people carries a genetic variant that makes them more likely to develop an AI. Some doctors may be comfortable letting patients think it ends with genetics. However, environmental triggers that enter our body and mimic estradiol play a huge role in the actual activation of AI diseases. From my research, I firmly believe The Pill is to lupus as cigarettes are to lung cancer.

There are still doctors out there following in the footsteps of Dr. Bole. I contacted Dr. William V. Williams, Adjunct Professor of Medicine at the University of Pennsylvania, who said, "The evidence is clear that The Pill increases the risk women will develop autoimmune disease, and that it often worsens Lupus disease activity."

Listen to your body. If it tells you that something doesn't 'feel right' about your hormonal contraceptive, pay attention - even if your doctor acts like it's nothing (and especially, if he/she suggests anti-depressants as the solution). Trust your questions more than the answer.

CHAPTER 18

Multiple Sclerosis

As I write this, the top hit for the Google search, "birth control + multiple sclerosis" features the dangerously deceptive headline, "Birth Control May Lower MS Risk." The linked article begins, "Women who take birth control pills may be less likely to develop multiple sclerosis (MS) while they're on the pill, according to a new study."

The key phrase is 'while they're on the pill,' but we will come back to that in a moment. First, let's zoom out and look at the broader picture of MS as an autoimmune disease.

Birth Control and Multiple Sclerosis

In the case of multiple sclerosis, errant T cells attack the myelin sheath that protects neural pathways of the nervous system. In Chapter 15, we saw how the cytokine, interleukin-6 (IL-6) can cause depression, but scientists have also identified IL-6 as the messenger that triggers T cells to become pathogenic in MS. A recent study suggests that "cluster signaling" of IL-6 from the surface of dendritic cells could cause "the T cell to become highly aggressive and efficient in attacking its target antigen."

Two other recent studies established mechanisms for increased IL-6 production in birth control users. The first study observed increased synthesis of C-Reactive Protein (CRP), which elevated in direct correlation to IL-6. Separate studies have shown CRP levels in birth control users to be two to three times those of nonusers.

Another study demonstrated lower cortisol production in birth control users, which led to higher levels of IL-6, since cortisol normally regulates IL-6. While neither study proves a definitive link between hormonal contraceptives and MS, they certainly demonstrate how these synthetic hormones make the user's body more conducive to the disease.

Birth Control Helps My Symptoms

Before examining more evidence, let's discuss why The Pill seems to relieve MS symptoms. Hormonal contraceptives flood the body with synthetic estrogen, similar to the body's natural process during pregnancy. By convincing the body it's pregnant each month, the contraceptive prevents actual pregnancy.

During an actual pregnancy, the flood of estrogens improves acute MS attacks by 80 percent (nearly doubling the efficacy of the best drugs on the market.) With certain autoimmune diseases like MS, sex hormones appear to promote inflammation when they're at normal levels but dampen it at higher levels.

Consequently, the flood of estrogens from hormonal birth control mimics the relief of pregnancy, but with a couple of dramatic pitfalls. First, hormonal contraceptives are synthetic and don't contain Estriol (E3), a pregnancy-specific hormone that seems to have the most therapeutic benefit. Second, hormonal birth control suppresses ovarian hormone production. In other words, the endocrine system reacts to the influx of synthetic estrogens by decreasing production of natural estrogens. Finally, while birth control provides temporary relief, it actually disrupts the endocrine and immune systems, which creates devastating consequences for MS symptoms in the long run.

Multiple Sclerosis' Growing Gender Gap

You may wonder how all this talk of T cells and endocrine disruptors translates to actual women. Unfortunately, the results are just as you would suspect. Kaiser Permanente released a study in 2014 disclosing that women who had taken The Pill were 35 percent more likely to develop multiple sclerosis than women who hadn't.

Relative to gender, multiple sclerosis has always been a discriminatory disease because of the way it engages with estrogen. However, all indicators point to a dramatic widening of the gender gap since the introduction of birth control pills. According to Gary Cutter PhD., professor of biostatistics at the University of Alabama, in 1940, twice as many women as men had multiple sclerosis. By 2000, four out of five MS patients were women. That's a 50 percent increase over each decade!

A report published in the *Neurology Journal* confirmed the increased gender gap as a global trend. After reviewing global epidemiological data, the researchers found that the female-to-male ratio was approximately 1.4 in 1955, and had jumped to 2.3 by the year 2000. Sreeram Ramagopalan, Ph.D., research fellow at University of Oxford, offered this commentary on the study:

"This intriguing epidemiological phenomenon warrants particular attention because the sex ratio of MS parallels MS incidence, and the increasing frequency of MS among females is a key driver of the increasing prevalence of this devastating disorder worldwide. <u>A change that occurs within a century is too short a time for a genetic cause. This suggests that environmental factor(s) are at work in a sex-specific manner.</u>"

Pardon me for pointing to the elephant in the room, but evidence has already mounted against one particular sex-specific environmental factor that's been influencing the rise in MS among women over the past 50 years.

CHAPTER 19

Crohn's Disease:
What's Wrong with Western Medicine

It's funny how clearly some mundane memories stick in your mind. I still recall the first time I took my car in for an instant oil-change. They hooked me with the promise to be out in under 10 minutes, and something about navigating my vehicle over the huge hole in the floor appealed to the little boy inside me. In fact, the entire experience was pretty pleasant… right up until the technician approached my window at the eight-minute mark.

"You're going to need a new valve soon, and your air filter is really dirty. Would you like me to replace these today?"

He was carrying the dirty filter and PCV valve as proof. I thought to myself, "They've been riding in a car engine. Of course, they're dirty!" After he told me the cost,

I politely declined. I'm not really a car guy, but I suspected I could get them cheaper elsewhere.

I'm skeptical anytime I know someone is trying to sell me something. That doesn't make me unique; it makes me human. That's why word-of-mouth advertising is so effective. If a friend (or even a stranger on Yelp) tells us something is great and we know they aren't being paid to say so, their opinion carries that much more value.

That air filter, though. It was nasty! So, I drove directly to a parts store, and it was indeed about half the cost. My inner imp felt justified.

A few thousand miles later I returned to the same shop for another oil change. (The sacrifices we make in the name of 'instant'). Imagine my surprise when the eight-minute interlude again featured the same air filter – the one I had just replaced. On the Scale of Betrayal, the technician was hardly Judas, but I still vowed never to take my car there again.

In my opinion, that's the definition of healthy skepticism, one that steers us clear of people who don't have our best interests in mind.

What's Behind the Message?

In the oil change shop, it's easy to spot the salesman's motivation, but in some scenarios, it's difficult to spot the salesman, much less his/her motivation.

That healthy skepticism may never be more absent than when we visit the doctor. Ironically, because of the odd paradigm within the medical industry, that is precisely when it should be at its sharpest. I can't think of another scenario where the consumer of the product relies so completely on someone else to make the purchase decision. Perhaps our skepticism is alleviated because we believe the physician has taken an oath to 'first do no harm.' However, about one out of every five medical students actually reports taking no oath at all.

With or without the oath, we, the consumer, will be the ones taking the treatment they prescribe. We will be the ones living with the consequences, good or bad. Given that those consequences are all too often chronic or deadly, we should absolutely question a doctor's reasoning and motivation.

Questioning Consensus

Crohn's Disease affects absorption on the surface of the intestine, which can diminish the effectiveness of hormonal birth control. Consequently, the prevailing consensus among doctors is to counter the effect Crohn's has on The Pill by switching the patient to a higher dosage. In the long run, this can be devastating.

Unfortunately, this reflects a pretty typical standard of practice for dealing with problems in the medical industry. You either increase the dosage, or you prescribe something 'off-label,' especially when it comes to The Pill. Hormonal contraceptives are prescribed off-label to treat everything from acne and irregular periods to PCOS and multiple sclerosis.

Doctors tend to think of prescribing off-label as being cutting edge. I once heard the lead investigator for a new drug trial say, "We all know the FDA lags behind the standard of practice." In her mind, I suppose the bureaucrats just can't keep up with all the fantastic uses they keep finding for drugs. But, think for a moment about what 'off-label' means. It means the prescribed drug hasn't been clinically proven safe or effective for this particular use. It means treatment by consensus, rather than sound science. Alarmingly, a recent study published in *Obstetrics and Gynecology* revealed that a full two-thirds of practices in their specialty were based on consensus rather than 'good and consistent scientific evidence.'

Proactive in the Wrong Direction

Recognizing the effects of Crohn's Disease on the intestine and boosting a young woman's birth control may seem very proactive, but it doesn't take into account the big picture. In fact, it's like admiring the mountainous road behind the Mona Lisa while missing her smile.

Surprisingly few doctors recognize that birth control could have actually triggered her disease in the first place, even though the number of Crohn's Disease cases has exploded since the introduction of birth control pills. In 2015, Harvard researchers conducted a massive study of nearly a quarter-million health records and discovered that women who took hormonal birth control for five years, more than tripled their risk of developing Crohn's Disease.

But really, it shouldn't have taken a major Harvard study for doctors to consider the link to irritable bowel disease. After all, nausea and upset stomach are among the most common complaints after starting birth control. Estrogen is known to modify permeability and inflammation of the gut, and synthetic estrogen's effect is unquestionably harmful. Interestingly, the same study found women who take hormone replacement therapy face a 74 percent increased risk of ulcerative colitis, another irritable bowel disease.

Nothing New Under the Sun

News outlets hailed the Harvard study as groundbreaking. Any health periodical worth its weight in feathers ran an article on the study's *new* findings. However, one only needs to read the study's references to see how little ground it broke.

Citations and the year they were published, include (Condensed titles): Regional enteritis: possible association with oral contraceptives, 1969; Small intestine disease and oral contraceptive agents, 1973; Intestinal complications during the use of oral contraceptives, 1976; Colonic Crohn's disease and use of oral contraception, 1984; The risk of oral contraceptives in the etiology of inflammatory bowel disease, 2008.

After a 1999 study recognized hormonal contraceptive use as a high-risk factor for a relapse in Crohn's disease, *Gut British Medical Journal* published evidence that not only supported these findings, but also demonstrated a significant change in gender ratio, the incidence of female diagnoses compared to males jumped dramatically after the introduction of birth control pills.

Ultimately, the Harvard study was a massive population-based study that did little more than confirm what researchers had known (or at least suspected) since 1969.

In his testimony at the Nelson Pill Hearings (1970), Dr. Philip Ball detailed how The Pill affects nearly every tissue in a woman's body, and then offered this food for thought:

"I believe that we physicians are so used to administering very potent medications to very serious disease problems, we have not really yet learned it is a totally different circumstance to administer powerful but nonessential drugs chronically to healthy young women, as is done in contraceptive pill administration... It is not sensible to say that birth control pills are safer than pregnancy – we don't prescribe pregnancy. The question is simply, are the pills safer than the diaphragm or safer than the foams or rubber prophylactics? And the answer is clearly no.
"We have had much talk in our land about preserving our environment or improving our quality of life or preventing pollution of our country. The administration of birth control pills...may be termed an internal pollution by chemicals [that will] interfere with a woman's quality of life."

Buyer Beware

Common sense *and* science tell us that hormonal contraceptives probably aren't a great idea for someone with Crohn's Disease (or someone with a family history of Crohn's). Yet, we have already seen that the consensus among doctors is to *increase* the dosage of synthetic estrogen for these patients.

How can this be? And, what does it have to do with a speedy oil change?

Clearly, physicians aren't receiving a commission or bonuses for prescribing drugs, but that's not to say they aren't influenced by pharmaceutical companies in much the same way the oil change technician was influenced by his employers. Let's consider these commonalities: training, incentives, and pressure to perform.

Training – Drug manufacturers begin exerting influence on medical professionals early in their academic careers. As unwitting students, young doctors-to-be are typically unaware of the biases that could be shaping the way they will approach their practices. Refer to Chapter 8, to see how Big Pharma exerts influence over their education from the early days of medical school and continue in perpetuity with required continuing medical education.

Incentives – Just for fun, watch an hour of television and don't skip the commercials. In fact, count them. What percentage do you think will be prescription drug commercials?

I know it sounds more nausea-inducing than fun, but here's the point. Big Pharma spends three billion dollars-per-year advertising to consumers. As you think about those ubiquitous commercials and how far three billion dollars goes, consider this – Big Pharma spends **eight times more** on marketing directly to healthcare professionals, $24 billion annually.

The Food and Drug Administration, American Medical Association, and (PhRMA) Pharmaceutical Research and Manufacturers of America have all established guidelines and regulations in an attempt to limit gifts from the drug industry to healthcare professionals. The thought is that strictly limiting gifts will eliminate the influence drug companies have over those who write the scripts. Small gifts like a pharma sales rep bringing lunch to the doctor's staff on Tuesday couldn't possibly motivate him/her to prescribe more of their drug, right?

A recent study published in *JAMA Internal Medicine* found that, indeed, even a single $20 meal sponsored by a drug company can influence a doctor's prescribing habits, and the impact increases with each meal. According to NBC News:

> "Those who got four or more meals relating to the four drugs [in the study] prescribed Crestor nearly twice as often as doctors who didn't get the free meals; Bystolic more than five times as often, Benicar more than four times as often and Pristig 3.4 times as often."

These small gifts translate to a huge return on investment. The study found that when a drug company spends $13 on a doctor, they see 94 additional days of prescriptions for brand-name anticoagulants and an additional 107 days for brand-name drugs.

The Centers for Medicare and Medicaid Service track industry payments to healthcare professionals, and have made their database accessible to the public. You can discover if your physician receives payments from pharmaceutical companies and, if so, how much, by visiting: https://openpaymentsdata.cms.gov. ProPublica also created an interesting search tool using the same data, which you can utilize by visiting https://projects.propublica.org/docdollars/.

Pressure to Perform – You may feel happy for Joe Mechanic when he gets Employee of the Month for selling the most air filters, but how would you feel about drug companies tracking your doctor's performance? In fact, that's exactly what's happening.

Pharmaceutical companies buy physician prescribing data from companies like IMS Health. These weekly lists track every prescription written by healthcare professionals in the United States. Physician and patient names aren't included, but each prescription does include the doctor's Drug Enforcement Administration ID number. Interestingly, the American Medical Association makes about $20 million per year selling the master file of its physician database, which includes their DEA number.

By combining these two databases, the drug companies can see precisely how frequently each doctor prescribes their drug compared to the competition. Then, the sales reps can tailor their pitch and the amount of pressure to apply to each doctor.

Most doctors seem to realize that the gifts and pressure are influential but think that they are immune. Shannon Brownlee offered this perspective:

> "Most physicians make 'I'm OK, you're not' assumptions about their profession's susceptibility to such tactics. In one survey, 61 percent of the residents at the University of California, San Francisco Medical Center reported that they themselves are unmoved by drug company gifts. But when asked if they thought their colleagues were swayed, 84 percent said yes."

Signs of their influence over healthcare professionals are everywhere. How else would you explain the plethora of off-label prescriptions? Does it seem reasonable that seven out of ten people you meet today are taking a prescription, and 20 percent of them are taking at least five prescriptions?!

CHAPTER 20

Hair Was a Musical
Hair Loss Is a Drama

Once you become familiar with the wide variety of side effects linked to birth control, you begin to see them everywhere. Daily revelations paint a clearer picture of the large price women pay in order to take The Pill.

While recently working on a Fashion Week event, I was reminded of a very common but seldom-mentioned side effect. The celebrity hairstylist on stage caught my attention when she turned off her clippers and asked the audience, "How many of you who have been cutting hair for more than five years have noticed that women's hair is getting thinner and thinner each year?"

Nearly every hand went up across the vast sea of hairdressers in the audience. The hairstylist on stage continued, "I've been cutting hair for over 20 years, and let me tell you, this has been going on for a long time. Personally, I think it's all the processed foods we eat."

While our unhealthy diet can't be good for our hair, it's more likely the culprit at the root of this hair loss epidemic dates back to the beginning of hormonal birth control.

Hair... The Drama, Not the Musical

The script is the same as it was fifty years ago - only the players have changed.

Fade in on a young woman looking at the clump of hair in her brush. It reminds her that she needs to call maintenance to come and unclog her drain... again! She has spent so much time worrying about hair loss that she wonders if the stress from that has made the hair loss even worse. With each passing day, she grows more certain these follicle follies were first triggered by her hormonal birth control.

She confronts her doctor but he's quite confident that The Pill had nothing to do with it. She's at a loss... From that point, there are many alternate endings to the story. At best, the relationship between birth control and hair loss is a reluctant love story, but their relationship can't be denied. Well, it can be denied in much the same way President Clinton denied having 'relations with that woman.' You can get away with it for as long as no one acknowledges the evidence.

The Pattern of Female Baldness

Though doctors still frequently tell their patients that hormonal birth control has nothing to do with their hair loss, it is a symptom that has been acknowledged for decades in (of all places) the information pamphlet that comes with each package of the drug.

In fact, hair loss from contraceptives is largely responsible for the original women's health movement. Barbara Seaman and Alice Wolfson both wrote about their experience with hair loss after they started The Pill. Each woman was assured by multiple doctors that birth control wasn't causing her hair loss, and each came to the conclusion, on her own, that it was. The nonchalant attitude of their doctors inspired them to push back against a system that didn't seem to care.

Ms. Seaman joined the Women's Liberation Health Committee and subsequently wrote a popular book titled, *The Doctors' Case Against the Pill*. Her book inspired the Congressional hearings that questioned The Pill's safety. It was also at these hearings that Alice Wolfson became *the* original face of the women's health movement after she famously interrupted the hearings to question why 10 million women were being used as guinea pigs.

Ms. Seaman and Ms. Wolfson met at the hearings and became fast friends. Ms. Seaman later wrote about the hearings to say it brought the "uptown" and "downtown" feminists together on the issue of birth control safety. She and Ms. Wolfson would go on to found the National Women's Health Network. To this day, it is one of the nation's top women's health advocacy groups.

The First Clump

Concern about hair loss attributed to birth control dates back to at least 1965. That's when Dr. Rosamund Vallings wrote an inquiry to the *British Medical Journal* regarding some curious findings in her practice at a family planning clinic:

> "I have had three patients developing marked alopecia areata shortly after commencing oral contraceptives. I shall be interested to hear colleagues who have had similar findings."

Alopecia areata is an autoimmune disease (AI) in which the body's immune system attacks healthy hair follicles. In previous chapters on multiple sclerosis, lupus, and even depression, I outlined some of the key ways synthetic estrogens in birth control can trigger an AI. As further evidence, Aviva Romm M.D. stated in a recent interview, "Most doctors probably don't actually know the connection between autoimmune disease and birth-control pills, but it's not a subtle connection. It's a very clear connection. So some of these longer-term consequences can be completely missed…women who go on oral contraceptives have a dramatically higher chance of developing an autoimmune condition than women who don't — about a 30 to 50 percent increase."

Experiencing hair loss while on contraceptives doesn't necessarily mean you will be diagnosed with alopecia areata. As we will see in the next chapter, some hair loss can be caused by the effects of birth control on the thyroid. And of course, secondary factors such as a diagnosis of PCOS or endometriosis can exacerbate hair loss, as can other toxic medications – like the antidepressants that frequently accompany birth control.

It Should Come as No Surprise

In an article titled "Is Birth Control Making You BALD?," the Daily Mail recently interviewed hormone expert, Dr. Lara Briden about the epidemic affecting young women. Addressing some of the frequently blamed factors, Dr. Briden said, "'Previous generations of young women had the same genes and they also suffered iron deficiency, thyroid disease, PCOS and they dieted... The thing that has changed is that more women today use more hormonal birth control, and they've started it at a younger age."

In their story on the same subject, the Sydney Morning Herald interviewed David Salinger, the director of the International Association of Trichologists. He said, "The progesterone in some pills can have a male hormonal effect on the hair. If a female has a genetic tendency and she then takes something which has male hormonal effects, that can trigger the thinning. I'm seeing many, many women in their 20s and 30s getting this type of hair loss."

It is simply indefensible for any medical professional prescribing birth control not to be aware that hormonal contraceptives can cause dramatic hair loss. After all, it's a fact hairdressers have known for decades as indicated in this passage from Barbara Seaman's book, published in 1969:

> "Just as brassiere manufacturers are sure that more women are wearing C cups, many hairdressers are certain that the pill is making some of their clients lose hair. Indeed, just as the Food and Drug Administration includes breast changes among the

adverse reactions to the pill that must be listed by drug manufacturers, it includes loss of scalp hair as a possible adverse reaction that must be listed. This means that the agency has had enough reports of such reactions from doctors to take them seriously."

Looking back on it, I regret that I didn't track down the celebrity hairstylist to share some of these facts with her. If we can't count on doctors to share information about hair loss with their patients, maybe we can get the word out through their hair stylists.

CHAPTER 21

Thyroid, Liver, and Gallbladder

A lot of things baffle me about the medical industry's approach to birth control, but the one thing I've struggled with the most from the perspective of symptoms and disease has to do with the thyroid. For the life of me, I can't see how any doctor could prescribe The Pill to a patient and not be concerned about the effect it has on her thyroid.

The most frequent side effects experienced by women on birth control precisely parallel the symptoms of hypothyroidism: weight gain, water retention, constipation, irregular spotting, decreased libido, high cholesterol…

I believed one would have to be willfully blind not to see the connection. Then, I learned about another type of blindness in Daniel Kahneman's book, *Thinking, Fast and Slow*.

Blind to Hypothyroidism

Kahneman won a Nobel Prize for his seminal work in behavioral economics. In the book, he describes numerous ways our minds process information and the, sometimes illogical, ways we respond to particular situations. A couple of the cognitive processes he details could help explain why doctors tend to overlook birth control's effect on the thyroid.

First, what the author calls "a general 'law of least effort' [that] applies to cognitive as well as physical exertion.' He says we have a laziness built into our nature, and once we learn a skill, we utilize fewer regions of the brain and consume less energy when we perform the task. Consequently, we are less engaged.

The second factor has to do with attention. Kahneman explains, "When waiting for a relative at a busy train station, for example, you can set yourself at will to look for a white-haired woman or a bearded man, and thereby increase the likelihood of detecting your relative from a distance." However, by focusing your attention on spotting this relative, you will miss other details – and not just the mundane.

To demonstrate just how focused we can become on a task, he cites the Invisible Gorilla study, which achieved notoriety beyond the realms of behavioral science because it seems so impossibly absurd:

> "[The researchers] constructed a short film of two teams passing basketballs, one team wearing white shirts, the other wearing black. The viewers of the film were instructed to count the number of passes made by the white team, ignoring the black players.

This task is difficult and completely absorbing. Halfway through the video, a woman wearing a gorilla suit appears, crosses the court, thumps her chest, and moves on. The gorilla is in view for 9 seconds. Many thousands of people have seen the video, and about half of them do not notice anything unusual. It is the counting task - and especially the instruction to ignore one of the teams – that causes the blindness. No one who watches the video without the task would miss the gorilla."

Likewise, if a new patient, who hadn't recently started on The Pill, presented the same symptoms, no doctor would miss the warning signs of a hypoactive thyroid.

Focus on You

Doctors, through their training and experience, are intimately familiar with the common, less significant side effects of hormonal birth control. So when a patient develops these complications soon after starting The Pill, skilled doctors believe it to be normal. They may suggest the symptoms will go away with time or may choose to prescribe a different formulation.

Since they already know the source of the symptoms, the solution seems reasonable. It would be unnatural for them to consider the onset of a new disease caused by The Pill. After all, who keeps looking for the TV remote once they've found it?

This compartmentalization bias is precisely why a woman should trust her body more than the doctor when it comes to birth control. It's not a coincidence that many women's side effects resemble hypothyroidism (such as

Hashimoto's Thyroiditis), nor is it a coincidence that so many women develop a hyperactive thyroid (such as Grave's Disease) soon after they stop The Pill.

Thyroid Under Attack

A normally functioning thyroid's primary role is to produce two hormones known as T3 and T4. Produced in much smaller quantities, T3 is the active hormone, which regulates our energy, metabolism, and internal 'thermostat.' T4 could be thought of as T3 in waiting. It is produced in larger quantities so that it can be delivered throughout the body, where it will be converted to T3.

Each cell in the body contains receptors for the thyroid hormones. These receptors remove a single iodine molecule from the T4, transforming the T4 into active T3. Thanks to this little miracle of biochemistry repeating itself in every system of our body, the thyroid affects nearly every bodily function. Consequently, so does anything that disturbs that delicate balance.

Hormonal birth control creates myriad problems for the thyroid, beginning with the depletion of vital nutrients such as magnesium, selenium, zinc, and essential B Vitamins, like folate. The thyroid needs these essential nutrients, especially zinc and selenium, to convert T4 to T3. Unfortunately, no amount of supplements will help your body overcome this obstacle.

While depleting nutrients, birth control also elevates the production of Thyroid Binding Globulin (TBG). As the name suggests, this protein binds with thyroid hormones to carry them through the bloodstream but renders them unable to attach to cell receptors. Consequently, the body may try to compensate by overproducing T3 and T4, without actually increasing hormone activity. This could explain the mechanism that leads some women to develop Grave's Disease after stopping The Pill. Their TBG levels return to normal, but their body continues overproducing T3 and T4.

The Path to Long-term Fatigue

As we learned in Chapter 12, women taking hormonal contraceptives have also been shown to have up to a three-fold increase in C-Reactive Protein (CRP), a widely recognized inflammation marker. The liver kicks into overdrive producing CRP in response to the inflammation associated with the birth control. This inflammation serves as a double-whammy to the already struggling tandem of the thyroid and liver.

First, the inflammation makes your cell walls less responsive to all hormones. Second, it disturbs the process of deiodination, leading to the overproduction of another inactive hormone known as Reverse T3 (RT3). RT3 is literally the mirror image of T3, meaning the iodine molecule has been removed from the opposite side of the hormone.

RT3 competes with T3 for the same receptors. Since it is inactive, too much RT3 can leave you feeling lethargic, depressed, and sensitive to cold weather. You may begin to experience brain fog and hair loss. Your body responds by producing more cortisol in an attempt to boost your energy. If this continues for too long, it could lead to adrenal suppression and long-term fatigue.

Thyroid, Liver, and Gallbladder

Weighing on the Liver

So, what causes this inflammation in the first place? As the central organ in the metabolic process, the liver produces proteins, which break down fat and hormones to generate energy. When we overload the body with a flood of factory-produced, unnatural hormones, the liver becomes sluggish and inefficient. This sets off a toxic cascade of side effects that lead to inflammation, and could ultimately contribute to chronic illnesses such as heart disease, cancer, and autoimmune disease.

The National Institutes of Health was concerned about hormonal birth control's effect of the endocrine system from the very early days. When Dr. Philip Corfman, the Director of the Center for Population Research, testified at the Nelson Pill Hearings on behalf of the NIH, he warned that The Pill decreased the liver's ability to change and dispose of certain chemicals, even reducing its ability to excrete bile.

Their studies from the 1960s showed that up to 40 percent of women on oral contraceptives experienced some changes in thyroid function. They made the connection that this had also contributed to changes in adrenal gland function, citing increased cortisol levels. Reading from the NIH report he helped author, Dr. Corfman said:

"Although it is not yet possible to draw definite conclusions about their effect on the health of women and infants, the use of these agents warrants close observation and surveillance. Effects of special concern include alterations in carbohydrate metabolism, the character and distribution of lipids, liver function, protein metabolism, and the development of hypertension as well as alterations of endocrine function."

Congress followed up on the hearings with a special report issued in 1978. Beyond concerns addressed in the original hearings, the new Congressional Report discussed more hepatic complications associated with The Pill, including the 'greatly increased risk' of developing an otherwise rare form of benign liver tumor known as hepatocellular adenoma (HCA). Studies at that time showed that women who had taken The Pill for eight years were 500 times more likely to develop HCA, with four percent of those becoming cancerous.

Good News First

The good news is that many of the side effects of hormonal birth control are reversible if you stop taking them soon enough. Not every person who experiences symptoms of a hypoactive thyroid will develop Hashimoto's Thyroiditis. While environmental factors are pivotal in triggering the development of this chronic disease, you must also be genetically predisposed in order to be susceptible to Hashimoto's, or any other AI for that matter.

The bad news is that a <u>LOT</u> of people are genetically predisposed to Hashimoto's Thyroiditis. In fact, it is considered the most common autoimmune disease, at 46 cases per 1,000. An estimated 20 million Americans have some sort of thyroid disease, and Hashimoto's Thyroiditis makes up about 90 percent of those with hypoactive thyroids.

Little, But Not Insignificant

Researchers in the early 1970s began to notice that women taking hormonal birth control also experienced an increased risk of developing gallbladder disease. They initiated a study, which confirmed a biochemical basis for their observation. It demonstrated that there is significantly more cholesterol in a woman's gallbladder bile while she is on birth control.

Given that cholesterol stones make up nearly 80 percent of all gallstones, subsequent studies successfully demonstrated that synthetic estrogens and progestins play critical roles in the development of gallstones - a fact that could have severe consequences for a woman's health during her reproductive years. Indeed, women in their 30s are up to five times more likely to develop gallstones than their male counterparts, but that gender disparity begins to level out as we move out of the reproductive years.

Naysayers might argue that a woman's natural feminine hormones already make her more susceptible to gallstones, and there appears to be some truth to that argument. However, in 1993, researchers culled the information from 25 epidemiological studies and found that women who had taken birth control were 36 percent more likely to develop gallstones than women who had never taken it.

Not coincidentally, the number of cholecystectomies (surgery to remove the gallbladder) have been growing consistently year-to-year, and those numbers are likely to increase at an even greater pace in the near future with the introduction of Yaz and Yasmin, today's most popular birth control brands. Hitting the market in 2001, this new generation of pill contains the progestin, drospirenone, which has been found to increase a woman's chance of gallbladder disease by another 20 percent over previous formulas of birth control. Scientists say that drospirenone not only increases the amount of cholesterol in her bile, but it also decreases the gallbladder's movement — making conditions very favorable for gallstones to develop. Bayer, which manufactures both drugs, denies there is any proof of a link to their product. Nevertheless, to date, they have agreed to pay over $21 million to settle thousands of gallbladder-related lawsuits.

CHAPTER 22

Something in the Water

In early 2016, the Associated Press rolled out an alarming story about the municipal water supplies of several major U.S. cities containing relatively high concentrations of numerous prescription drugs. While the implications of the report extended beyond estrogen, it was the first time many Americans considered how far-reaching the contraceptive and endocrine disrupting consequences could be.

However, this wasn't news to environmental scientists. They had been on the trail of synthetic estrogens in our drinking water for over twenty years.

Tracking the Trace Elements

Toxicologists traditionally measure contaminants in water at levels in the parts-per-million. Elements that existed in parts-per-billion and parts-per-trillion have always been considered trace elements, which were thought to be so diluted that they would pose no real danger. Consequently, there are no regulations for contamination at these lower levels. Unfortunately, with the potency of synthetic estrogens, the threat is already very real once the concentration reaches levels in the parts-per-trillion.

Dr. David Norris, a Professor in the Department of Integrative Physiology at the University of Colorado-Boulder, has devoted fifty years of his life to studying these 'Stealth Pollutants' in our waterways. More on his work in a moment, but first, he says the best way to visualize how little estrogen it takes to begin disrupting the ecosystem is to imagine taking a pinch of salt and dropping it into an Olympic-sized pool. That is the concentration that begins to take its toll on vertebrate animals (Spoiler alert: That includes us).

The new millennium has ushered in a slow awakening in the scientific community about the dangers of hormonal contraceptives as a pollutant to those who encounter it both directly and indirectly. The World Health Organization classified hormonal contraceptives as Group 1 Carcinogens in 2005. While the risk may be most significant for the women who choose to take hormonal contraceptives each day, they clearly aren't the only ones in harm's way.

Consider this. A conservative estimate of 13 million women in the US take some form of hormonal contraceptive each day. Ethinyl estradiol, the synthetic hormone used in these drugs, has a biological activity about 100 times that of our natural hormones. In order to effectively prevent pregnancy, these molecules cannot break down in stomach acid, meaning they pass through the body virtually unchanged. Consequently, 13 million women flush these powerful chemicals into the sewage system every day.

Perhaps it isn't surprising then, that when a team from the University of Pittsburgh took extracts from catfish living downstream from sewage plants along the Allegheny and Monongahela rivers and exposed them to estrogen-sensitive breast cancer cells, the cancer began to multiply dramatically. However, not all of the consequences scientists are identifying could have been so easily predicted.

The Pill: It's Not Just for Women Anymore

In 1993, Scottish and Danish researchers published a report in the British Medical Journal, *The Lancet*, with the attention-grabbing announcement that we now live in a "Sea of Estrogens." They claimed that synthetic chemicals in the environment were mimicking natural estrogen, which was having a deleterious effect on male fetuses in the womb. They pointed to environmental pollutants like PCBs, detergents, dioxins, soy, and oral contraceptives. The media mostly reported on the other chemicals while downplaying The Pill, despite it being such a prolific and potent synthetic chemical explicitly designed for the purpose of mimicking natural estrogen in the body.

The very next year environmental scientists, led by John Sumpter, announced that male fish in 28 rivers across Britain were being 'feminized' by pollutants. *The Independent* reported that Professor Sumpter was studying fish because their reproductive systems are so similar to humans. Anything that disrupts the semen production in the two testes of a fish could likely have a similar impact on men.

The article goes on to say that the Department of the Environment, which funded the research, told scientists not to reveal the names of the affected rivers for fear of causing panic. I can only surmise that the desire to prevent panic must also explain how the following dubious statement made it into the article, "The contraceptive pill is not thought to be responsible for the oestrogens in sewage effluent because women excrete its hormones in a biologically inactive form that has no effect on fish."

Environmental Pollutants

However, in 2002, Susan Jobling of Brunel University focused the attention squarely on hormonal birth control. Her team demonstrated that fish populations crashed in areas downstream of effluent from sewage plants located along tributaries feeding the Thames River. And, Jobling wasn't shy about connecting the dots to make this a human problem as well.

Charles Tyler, a member of her team from Exeter University, explained:

"Synthetic oestrogen, ethanol oestradiol, is exquisitely potent at very, very low concentrations, between 50 and 100 times as potent as natural oestrogen.

"The level at which we can measure the effects in fish are below the levels which we can detect the chemical in drinking water, so we cannot be sure that some of these compounds, even at very low concentrations, are not getting into our drinking water."

Based on this research, the United Kingdom's Department of the Environment finally had enough evidence to take action and classify hormonal contraceptives as environmental pollutants in 2004. In 2012, the European Union proposed action that would require municipalities to upgrade existing sewage systems to remove these microbial pollutants. However, when the discussion turned to having pharmaceutical companies foot the bill, their powerful lobbyists went to work to have the proposal dismissed. As of this writing, over a decade later, they have still effectively delayed 'any decision on a regulatory environmental quality standard.'

Equal Opportunity Sterility

The Brits may have again been the first ones to address the issue, but this isn't just a European problem. It's a global problem, particularly in industrialized countries.

Dr. Karen Kidd, who led a seven-year Canadian lake study to examine the effects of this hormonal flushing, explains it this way, "Ethinyl estradiol has a two-carbon chain, which makes it more resistant to metabolism in our bodies, but also more resistant to degradation in the environment."

With her team, she calculated the concentrations of ethinyl estradiol (EE2) that would be released into the waterways via sewage coming from a city of 200,000 people, and she released that amount into a test lake each day. Her team witnessed an immediate feminization and transgendering of male fish, which resulted in the "near extinction" of the fathead minnow population. And, the consequences started their ascent up the food chain in a measurable way, specifically in the feminization of trout, mink frogs and green frogs.

What made Dr. Kidd's study so remarkable was that they were able to make a solid case for cause and effect. They had control group lakes. They were able to introduce a single variable into the test lake (EE2). And, even though the minnow populations neared extinction, they rebounded as soon as the researchers stopped adding EE2 to the lake.

Study after study drew the correlation between estrogens in the water and the feminization of fish, including a 2006 study from the United States Geological Survey. Their team conducted tests on smallmouth bass in the Shenandoah and Monocacy Rivers and found that more than 80 percent of all the male bass living in these waterways were growing eggs in their testes.

Real World Meets the Lab

Starting in 2000, the aforementioned Dr. David Norris and his team began studying fish populations relative to the sewage treatment plants of three major Colorado cities: Denver, Boulder, and Colorado Springs. At each municipality, they set up a location just upstream from where the effluent was released, and another just downstream. The fish in the upstream locations enjoyed a balanced 1:1 female-to-male sex ratio. Downstream there were five female fish for every one male, and 20 percent of the reduced male population demonstrated intersex characteristics, such as eggs in their testes and the presence of Vitellogenin, an egg yolk protein normally found only in fertile females.

A few years into the study, the Boulder Water Works plant was forced to upgrade their facilities because of high ammonia levels in their processed water. The $50-million upgrade happened to also significantly reduce the number of estrogenic chemicals passing through the facility. Much like the results found at the Canadian test lakes, after the estrogenic compounds were removed, the downstream fish populations in Boulder began to normalize.

This is important to those of us further up the food chain because it demonstrates that advances in treatment technologies can be a useful tool in the fight against these stealth pollutants, but is it enough to keep us from drowning in this sea of estrogens?

Of Fish and Men

Scientists continue to argue about just how clear and how present the danger to men really is, but recent studies suggest the answer is very clear and very present. A 2017 study out of Hebrew University and Mount Sinai medical school found that sperm counts in human men have dropped by more than half since 1973. The study inspired a feature story in GQ magazine, where one of the lead investigators from the study offered this dire warning, "We should hope for the best and prepare for the worst, and that is the possibility that we will become extinct."

For more answers about what's happening to sperm counts, GQ's author, Daniel Noah Halpern, traveled to Copenhagen to meet one of the trailblazers in the field,

Dr. Niels E. Skakkebaek, one of the investigators from the "Sea of Estrogens" study. According to Mr. Halpern, "Skakkebaek first suspected something was going wrong in the late '70s, when he treated an infertile patient with an abnormality in the cells of the testes that he had never seen before. When he treated a second man with the same abnormality a few years later, he began to investigate a connection."

Because of the dramatic rise in these types of cases over a relatively short timeframe, Dr. Skakkebaek theorized that male fetuses are being exposed to environmental factors in the womb, which are antagonistic to their male sex hormones and are affecting their reproductive development. Depending on when the fetus is exposed to these harmful chemicals, the effect, which he calls testicular dysgenesis syndrome (TDS), can play out in numerous ways, such as abnormal genitalia, testicular cancer, and poor semen quality.

The effects of TDS parallel those of men whose mothers were given forms of the earliest marketed synthetic estrogen, diethylstilbestrol (DES), decades ago. You will recall from Chapter 6, DES had been banned for use by poultry farmers as a growth hormone because of its carcinogenic properties, but it was being prescribed off-label for pregnant women to prevent miscarriages.

Dr. Skakkebaek contends in his work that we find ourselves already in the midst of a fertility crisis. He writes, "Paradoxically, the total number of people might still be increasing for a couple of decades in spite of the birth rates below replacement level, because elderly people who now live longer more than compensate for… the fewer children."

CHAPTER 23

How Do We Fix This Problem?

In recent years, more people have become aware of the dangers of synthetic estrogens. We avoid plastics with BPA because of their estrogenic properties. We happily pay more for organic fruit, and for meat and dairy products that promise "No Artificial Hormones." But, these valiant attempts to cut back on our synthetic estrogen exposure are about as effective as ordering a diet cola with our Super-Sized meal and hoping to lose weight.

The problem is that estrogen exposure comes from all directions. For example, even if you invest in a reverse osmosis system to treat the drinking water in your home, there are other ways the synthetic estrogens from sewage can find their way back to you. Biosolids from wastewater treatment plants are also saturated with birth control estrogens, and more than half of this polluted sludge is sold to agricultural entities for fertilizer. Which means, the synthetic hormones end up in our food supply.

Improving sewage plants so that they are equipped to remove these stealth pollutants seems like an obvious place to start. However, as we saw with the examples in Boulder and the United Kingdom, these upgrades are cost prohibitive and completely unrealistic for most municipalities. Perhaps a better place to start would be with the most potent and pervasive of these stealth pollutants. As it turns out, in our current political climate, suggesting there are options other than hormonal birth control may be even more daunting than retooling our sewage systems?

Touching the Third Rail

Ironically, Dr. Kidd and Dr. Norris, whose work we explored in Chapter 22, are both quick to point out that they aren't against The Pill, nor do they think women should stop taking hormonal birth control. Imagine a researcher who discovered the dangers of second-hand smoke feeling compelled to assure the public that they didn't want to take away their right to smoke - not only that - imagine the researcher encouraging them to keep smoking.

If we want to be honest – intellectually, scientifically, and politically, we have to be willing to say The Pill is dangerous, and it's affecting all of us. There are better, safer options. And, we need to dramatically reduce the quantity of hormonal contraceptives being taken sooner rather than later!

How Do We Fix This Problem?

With the overwhelming evidence against The Pill, you would think this would be an easy agreement to reach. However, The Pill holds a sacred position in our culture. It's been made an icon of sexual freedom and women's liberation. Although there are numerous contraceptive and family planning options with fewer complications, the narrative has been defined in such a way that 'birth control' equals 'The Pill' equals 'Women's Rights.' This is incredibly fortunate for the pharmaceutical companies because any 'attack' on their product can be spun as an attack on Women's Rights.

In her book, Sweetening The Pill, Holly Grigg-Spall details how there is not only social pressure on young women to take hormonal contraceptives, but that the estrogens may actually be addictive. With so many valid alternatives, she suggests that the pharmaceutical companies are the only ones benefitting from this scenario, while individual women are the ones assuming the risk to their health.

She describes a new breed of feminists who look at The Pill from a different perspective. She writes:

"Radical menstruation activists believe that the act of stopping and hiding our periods with hormonal contraceptives and sanitary products is a mark of corporate ownership over our bodies. To them, being open and honest about menstruation and critical of the prescription of hormonal contraceptives is an important element of establishing an identity that is independent of the pressures of consumerism. They encourage women to separate out what they want, feel and like from what they are pressured to choose and from there begin to construct their selves outside of the boundaries of what they are told is appropriate."

She penned a follow-up article for the website, Hormones Matter about questions she had received from women who were concerned that her rejection of The Pill could be seen as an attack on women's rights:

"The answer [is] to seize the means of reproduction. Dependence on decision makers, or making choices from fear, is not the way forward. What we needed then, as we need now, is a birth control rebellion.
"One way to take back power from those who would deny, bully or browbeat you is to not need what they are fighting over."

There is simply too much evidence mounting against hormonal birth control to allow politics to justify inaction. Whether it be The Pill, a patch, ring, injection, or IUD, it isn't hyperbole to say that this issue is shifting the balance of nature. If we can't defend the truth because we fear how it might impact our political ideology, we risk becoming sycophants. And then, we risk becoming extinct.

For the Benefit of the Woman

Finding a global solution to deal with hormonal pollution is imperative, but by turning our focus downstream (literally and figuratively), we lose sight of the internal pollution suffered by the millions of victims who expose themselves directly to large doses of these potent chemicals each day.

Make no mistake, these patients are victims of a medical system controlled by the pharmaceutical industry. At best, these women make their decision based on minimally informed consent. Many don't even make the decision; they just trust that the doctor knows best.

The rare physician who doesn't hand out birth control like candy may warn his/her patients of minor side effects but typically mitigates even these by then telling her that her body just needs to adjust. Let's not forget this is the very same medical industry, which not so long ago told us smoking cigarettes was good for us.

Closing Arguments

In my conversations with women who have begun to doubt The Pill, it seems like there are two phrases that most frequently come from professionals trying to reassure them. They often succeed in assuaging fears, but they are very deceptive. I would like to address each of these in a sort of closing argument for my case against The Pill.

"Benefits versus risks" – Whenever a patient reads that The Pill has been linked to a specific disease, there will invariably be a quote from an expert assuring her, "The benefits still outweigh the risks."

The introduction of The Pill shifted many paradigms in this country, but perhaps the biggest shift came in the interpretation of "benefit to risk." We covered this in detail in Chapter 7, but I think it's worth highlighting again. Anytime you read 'the benefits still outweigh the risks' when associated with The Pill, remember the doctors at the Nelson Pill Hearings who proclaimed that the risk of overpopulation was so great that we now needed to consider the benefit to society versus the risk to the individual woman. The Pill was deemed so important to society that the men in power twisted the 'benefit-to-risk' paradigm in order to get it approved and distributed as a mass population experiment unlike any in history – before or since.

This is an epic and consequential shift to the paradigm because apparently the risk of cancer, stroke, heart disease, depression, hair loss, infertility, multiple sclerosis, lupus, diabetes, and scores of other autoimmune diseases to the individual woman isn't enough to outweigh the balance of the benefit to society in the eyes of those controlling the message.

"It's genetic" – Here's another scenario I've encountered numerous times, especially related to autoimmune disease. A young woman will begin to connect the dots, realizing that her disease symptoms either began shortly after she started on birth control, or that the symptoms were compounded by it. She receives some information, which confirms that other women have had a similar experience. She schedules an appointment with her doctor, who then convinces her that the disease is genetic. She leaves the appointment thinking she got it all wrong in blaming The Pill.

It's true that all autoimmune diseases have a basis in genetics. You have to be genetically predisposed to acquire the disease, but this isn't an either/or proposition. Environmental factors are key to triggering autoimmune diseases, and studies on identical twins have shown that hormonal birth control is a major factor in the triggering process. Therefore, it's a complete fallacy for a doctor to say, "The Pill didn't cause your disease because that disease is genetic."

How Do We Fix This Problem?

Spread the News

In the first chapter, I shared a question with you that ultimately led me to write this book, "When you're privy to information about The Pill, and you know most women haven't been given that information, does your responsibility change?"

I think it does. I hope the information I've shared in these pages will motivate you to action – whatever form that action takes - maybe it's just loaning this book to a family member.

If you finally found the answers to questions you had about your autoimmune disease or some other illness, I hope this book brought you comfort, and I hope you're encouraged to spread the word. The genetic nature of your disease means it's even more imperative that you share this information with the young women in your family. In being proactive and warning them about The Pill, you can save them from future suffering, because they are unquestionably at risk!

If we've learned anything from the past five decades, it's that we can't trust the medical industry at-large to be honest about the dangers of birth control. By taking it upon ourselves and informing the younger generation *before* they start hormonal birth control, we will empower them to make truly informed decisions about their reproductive health.

Consider becoming political. This is a non-partisan plea. It doesn't matter if you vote red or blue, and it doesn't matter if your Senator or Representative sits on the opposite side of the aisle. When it really comes down to it, hormonal birth control and women's health transcend politics – or at least they should. It's easy to lose sight of that in today's political climate.

Much of the foundation for this book came from the Nelson Pill Hearings – which were 50 years ago. Sadly, the situation hasn't improved since those first generation pills. In fact, in some regards, it's gotten worse.

Write to Congress and tell them it's time for more hearings. It's time to hold the drug companies accountable for the sad state of women's health.

It doesn't serve you or me – it doesn't serve the Republicans or Democrats to have women suffering from chronic ailments or even dying in the name of The Pill. In the end, it only serves the bottom line of the drug companies. Maybe that's what they really mean when they keep telling us 'the benefits still outweigh the risks.'

Resources & Further Reading

The Doctors' Case Against The Pill
by Barbara Seaman

The Greatest Experiment Ever Performed on Women
by Barbara Seaman

Pregnant or Dead
by Dr. Harold Williams

Sweetening The Pill
by Holly Grigg-Spall

Reproductive Rights and Wrongs
by Betsy Hartmann

The Pill: An Alarming Report
by Morton Mintz

D.E.S. – The Bitter Pill
by Robert Meyers